ASSESSING VITAL FUNCTIONS ACCURATELY

ASSESSING VITAL FUNCTIONS ACCURATELY

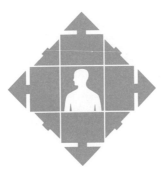

Nursing79 Books
Intermed Communications, Inc.
Horsham, Pennsylvania

NURSING80® BOOKS

Publisher: Eugene W. Jackson
Editorial Director: Daniel L. Cheney
Graphics Director: John Isley
General Manager: T. A. Temple

NURSING SKILLBOOKTM SERIES
SERIES EDITOR: Patricia S. Chaney
Clinical Editor: Barbara McVan, RN
Book Editor: Emily Heine
Assistant Editor: Avery Rome
Copy Editor: Patricia A. Hamilton
Production Manager: Bernard Haas
Production Assistants: David C. Kosten, Margie Tyson
Designers: Maggie Arnott and John Isely
Artists: Bob Arufo, Robert Renn, Elizabeth Clark, and Sandra Simms

Divider assemblages by Jack Gregory; photographs by Seymour Mednick
Anatomical drawings on dividers courtesy of GRAY'S ANATOMY, 29th
Edition, © 1973, Lea and Febiger, Philadelphia, Pa.
Slides of skin conditions courtesy Edward Glifort, Department of Dermatology,
University of Pennsylvania, and Gerald Pearlman, Skin and Cancer Hospital,
Temple University Health Sciences Center.

Library of Congress cataloging in publication data:

Main entry under title:

ASSESSING VITAL FUNCTIONS ACCURATELY
"Nursing Skillbook series"
Includes index.
1. Physical diagnosis.   2. Vital signs — Measurement.
3. Nursing.
RT48.A85 1977B   616.07'54   78-24419
ISBN 0-916730-05-0

CONTENTS

AUTHORS

Major Nancy Adams is the critical care coordinator at the William Beaumont Army Medical Center in El Paso, Texas. Her extensive medical background includes staff, ICU, and E.R. nursing.

Marie Scott Brown is assistant professor at the University of Colorado School of Nursing in Denver. She graduated from Marquette University in Milwaukee and the University of Colorado. She coauthored the book, PEDIATRIC PHYSICAL DIAGNOSIS FOR NURSES.

Roberta Erickson is assistant professor at the University of Portland's School of Nursing in Oregon. She has worked as an ICU staff nurse at the Good Samaritan Hospital and Medical Center in Portland, Oregon, and as an instructor in medical/surgical nursing at the School of Nursing of the University of Washington in Seattle. Ms. Erickson earned a BSN at the University of Arizona and a MSN at Wayne State University.

Carolyn Jarvis is an instructor in the school of nursing at the University of Missouri. Mrs. Jarvis has a BSN degree from the University of Iowa and an MSN degree from Loyola University in Chicago. She has worked in the thoracic ICU at the University of Missouri Medical Center and as a practitioner-teacher at Rush Presbyterian-St. Luke's Medical Center in Chicago. Her articles have appeared in SOCIOLOGY OF HEALTH CARE.

Marion Johnson is a clinical specialist and assistant professor at the University of Iowa Hospitals and College of Nursing. She has a BSN degree from the College of St. Theresa in Winona, Minnesota, and an MSN degree from Case-Western Reserve University in Cleveland. Ms. Johnson's articles have appeared in NURSING CLINICS OF NORTH AMERICA, AMERICAN JOURNAL OF NURSING, and NURSING DIGEST.

Louise Juliani is a clinical nurse specialist at the University of Wisconsin Hospitals in Madison. She earned a BSN at the University of Wisconsin and a MSN at Boston University. She serves as a member of the Wisconsin Kidney Foundation and the A.N.A.

Kathleen Marchiondo is a staff nurse in the intensive care unit of St. Joseph's Hospital, Albuquerque, New Mexico. After earning a BS degree in nursing from the University of New Mexico, Mrs. Marchiondo worked at Bernillillo County Medical Center, for part of that time as head nurse on a surgical specialties unit. She has published in PERSPECTIVES IN PSYCHIATRIC CARE.

Helen Morrow is assistant professor at Seattle Pacific University. An MN from the University of Washington, Mrs. Morrow lectures to RN inservice education groups on the blood-gas problems most often encountered in daily practice.

Mary Alexander Murphy is an assistant professor in the pediatric nurse practitioner program at the University of Colorado in Denver. She is a frequent contributor to *NURSING77* and on its advisory board.

Mary Delaney Naumoff is assistant professor in the health nurse clinician program at Wayne State University. She earned her BSN at Mercy College of Detroit and her MSN at Wayne State University.

Annalee Oakes, an assistant professor at Seattle Pacific University, uses her understanding of blood gases not only in clinical practice but also in student teaching. Mrs. Oakes holds a BSN and an MA from the University of Washington and is a certified CCRN.

Lora B. Roach is assistant professor at Texas Woman's University, College of Nursing, in Dallas. Ms. Roach is a graduate of Parkland Hospital School of Nursing in Dallas and was awarded a BS and an MS from the University of Texas. A charter member of the Alpha Delta chapter of Sigma Theta Tau, she received the Nurse-of-the-Year Award in 1970 from District #4 of the Texas Nurses' Association.

Frances Storlie is a clinical specialist in cardiovascular nursing. A prolific writer, Mrs. Storlie has published NURSING AND THE SOCIAL CONSCIENCE, PRINCIPLES OF INTENSIVE CARE, and THE CARDIAC SURGICAL PATIENT.

Carol Margaret Taylor is assistant professor of medical/surgical nursing at Vanderbilt University School of Nursing in Nashville, Tennessee.

Sharon Wahl is an instructor in medical/surgical nursing at the University of Oregon. She has served as an instructor in neurological nursing at the University of Portland and has designed a continuing education course on perspectives in neurological nursing. Mrs. Wahl has a BSN degree from the University of Portland and an MSN degree from the University of Oregon.

Loy Wiley is a senior editor of *NURSING77*.

Edwina McConnell, RN, MSN, served as special consultant to this book. **Crystal McCollister, RN, Catherine C. Manzi, RN,** and **Hannelore Sweetwood, RN, BS,** contributed to the Skillchecks.

FOREWORD

AS RECENTLY AS 1940, nurses weren't permitted to take a patient's blood pressure. But in the past 3 decades our roles have changed drastically. Today we're not only measuring traditional vital signs such as blood pressure — we're also assessing patients with sophisticated tools such as electrocardiograms and intra-arterial catheters; advising patients on health matters; and initiating programs in patient education. And our role will continue to change. Nurses everywhere are asking for more than auxiliary or handmaiden status. Indeed, some argue that our role be expanded even further to include such functions as performing screening procedures, ordering a wide range of laboratory tests, performing minor surgery, even prescribing certain types of medications.

Does all of this intimidate me? No. In fact, I'm thrilled! Because it speaks of a rising consciousness of who nurses are, and what we can contribute. How much we can do, such as transferring a patient from a ward, or ordering specific laboratory tests, or initiating nursing interventions, will depend on the autonomy we have. For nurses who are properly prepared, intervention and autonomy go hand in hand. The move — however embryonic — against standing orders and treatment protocols proves again that we have the courage to share our vision of nursing's future.

Nurses everywhere seem keenly aware that their rights to independence and accountability rest on advanced preparation, skills, and knowledge. Many match their demands for expanded roles with a willingness to continue their education in community colleges, technical institutions, or universities. Others subscribe to a variety of professional journals, enroll in approved correspondence courses, or read books such as this one. In short, nurses are learning about — learning to perform — new procedures, learning to evaluate their patients and to intervene in their behalf. The wide range of topics making up this Skillbook attests to the scope and depth of nurses' desire to become experts in nursing care.

I dream that one day our expanded role will mean independent decision-making, total accountability, and patient-centered intervention — responsibilities for which many of us have been well prepared and thousands of our colleagues are preparing themselves. When all of our assessments, all of our decisions, all of our interventions are judged for their benefit to the patient, our roles will automatically expand. I believe this Skillbook can help us prepare for that time.

—FRANCES STORLIE, RN, MS, PHD
Assistant Professor
Cardiovascular Nursing
Graduate Program
Arizona State University

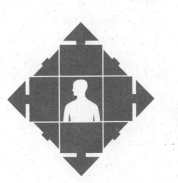

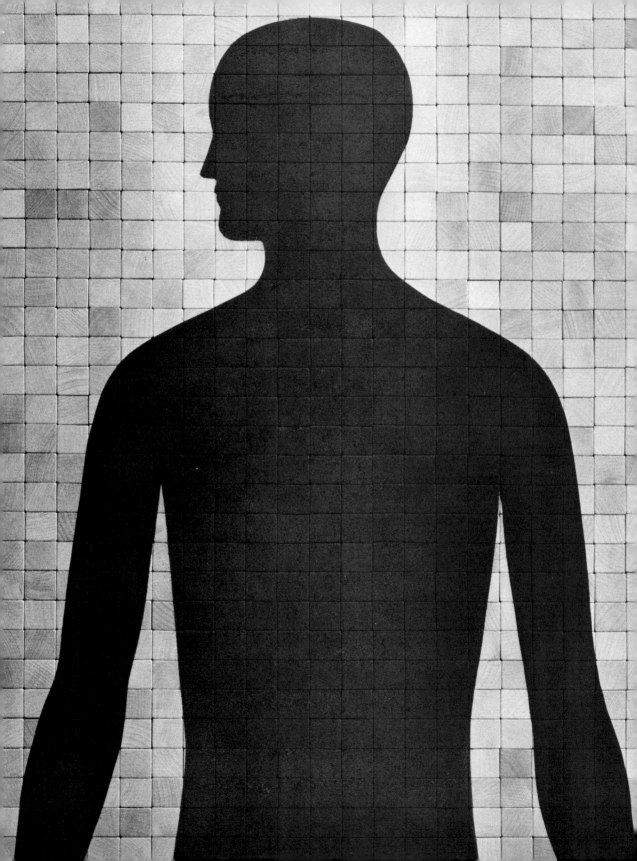

BEGINNING
WITH
BASICS

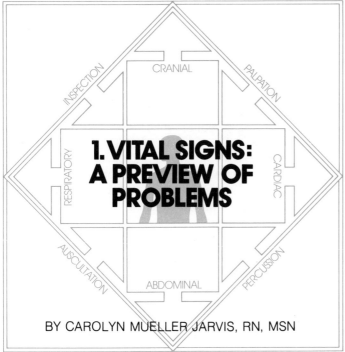

1. VITAL SIGNS: A PREVIEW OF PROBLEMS

BY CAROLYN MUELLER JARVIS, RN, MSN

YOU CAN LOOK at vital signs two ways. You can regard them as one more nursing chore, unthinkable to skip but meaning little — unless results are grossly abnormal, of course, when you sound the alarm and everybody comes rushing.

Or you can look at them a better way — not only as indicators of the patient's present condition, but also as critical signposts that can point ahead to trends and developments, good or bad, and to otherwise unsuspected pitfalls and needless complications.

Nobody is infallible, but I have learned that merely recording the temperature, pulse, respiration, and blood pressure is not enough. Only when I try to interpret all that these four sturdy guideposts can tell me do I know their meaning, what nursing measures the patient needs, or even when to call the doctor. We must be familiar with not one but all three parts — the signs, their meaning, and the measures to take.

How best to get and interpret these four clues to the body's state? You need a system for taking vital signs. You need a data base for each patient. And you need to remember that taking and assessing vital signs is a serial process, not a one-time affair. Only then do the results count for the most.

The system. Routine vital signs should be taken by the person caring for the patient during that shift rather than by someone assigned the task for the whole floor.

They should be taken in a systematic manner. For a complete picture, the data should be compared bilaterally. Once you have established your own way of doing it, unless there's some reason to change your routine for the sake of a particular patient, do it the same way every time. Otherwise you might omit something. And consistency will make you more sensitive to variation than will using a novel approach every time. Because, after all, variation — from the norm, from the patient's norm, and from the patient's last reading — is what vital signs are all about.

At the bedside, be aware of what your manner may imply despite your reassuring words. If you tell a patient he's fine but, wearing a furrowed brow, you take his blood pressure three or four times in a row and then call in another staff member to check your findings, that patient is going to be worried. Why not just tell him the truth: "Your blood pressure is up a little, so I am going to check it a few more times to see if there is a difference."

Data base. When you take vital signs, you're gathering facts for your data base. Know what's normal for your patient, and learn his vital signs from the previous shift. The more you know about the patient's vital signs, the more meaningful will be your data base for him. As early as you can, you'll want to interview the patient to learn how he perceives his state of health as well as to get his history.

A serial process. Gather vital signs as often as you think necessary. Don't wait for the next scheduled time if you suspect that a trend is developing. Establishing trends or comparing changes is much more meaningful than writing down one-time figures.

Interpretation. Take your data on the patient's vital signs and put it together with his diagnosis, lab tests, history, and charted records. Then analyze the information in terms of his complete health status including psychological and social behavior. Do you see any relationships among the data? Do you see any trends evolving? Are any of the abnormal vital signs you've found to be expected because of the patient's condition?

To analyze the data, you will need to know the normal range

of each vital sign, know the patient, know his own variations, and arrive at the meaning of it all. Only then can you make the best nursing assessment and work out the best nursing plan.

Temperature: Highs and lows

By what route do you take the temperature? The oral is possibly the most accurate. But if the patient has recently swallowed liquids or smoked, wait 15 minutes. And always leave the thermometer in place for 8 to 9 minutes. Axillary temperatures are safe and accurate for infants in a controlled environment. Use the rectal route when the others aren't practical for confused or comatose patients, or for those who can't close their mouths because of oxygen tubes, wired mandibles, or other facial handicaps. And then leave the thermometer in at least 2½ minutes.

How often should temperatures be checked? The answer, of course, depends on how often vital signs might be expected to change. In a medical or surgical unit timing will obviously be much more frequent than that in a chronic or psychiatric ward. As for the antiquated habit of waking your patients for a 6 a.m. check, one authority recommends this: Take temperatures routinely between 4 and 8 p.m., and check early morning temperatures only on patients who had a fever above 99.5° F. the previous evening, or on those who have had surgery the day before or will have it that day.

The normal oral range in a resting patient is 97.7° to 99.5° F. (36.5° to 37.5° C.). Rectal temperatures register 1° F. higher. Both are usually 1° to 2° F. lower in early morning than in late afternoon. Properly taken, these are core temperatures. But surface temperature can vary greatly with the temperature of the surrounding environment: It simply depends upon the amount of blood circulating in the skin.

When palpating for temperature, use the backs of your fingers, for the nerve endings there are more sensitive to subtle temperature changes. Another trick in finding local changes: Lay your fingers down, one hand on either side of the patient, leave them a minute, and then cross the placement of your hands. Any contrast will be apparent at once.

The body maintains a stable temperature by balancing heat production with heat loss through a thermostat or feedback mechanism in the hypothalamus of the brain. In illness or central nervous system disease or injury, the thermostatic

What is body temperature?

The body acquires heat through basal metabolism in the cells, muscle activity, and external sources (clothing, sunshine, hot liquids, etc.). It loses heat through radiation (about 60%), convection (12%), evaporation of perspiration (25%), and conduction (3%). Body temperature represents the balance between heat gain and heat loss.

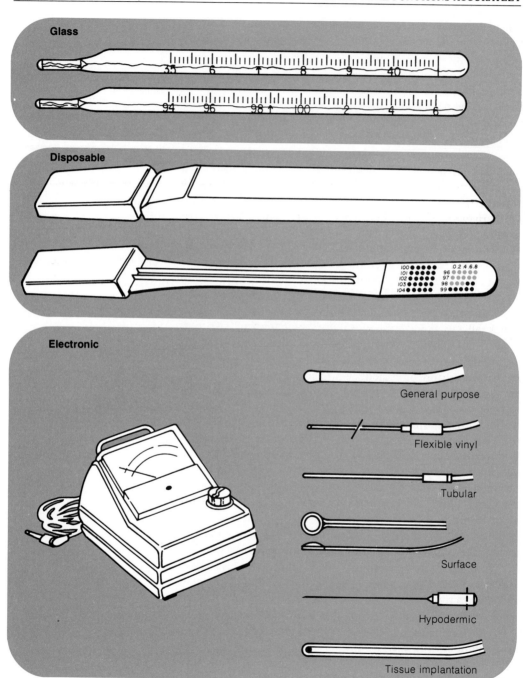

Glass

Disposable

Electronic

General purpose

Flexible vinyl

Tubular

Surface

Hypodermic

Tissue implantation

function may be scrambled. Pyrogens secreted by toxic bacteria in pneumonia, phlebitis, meningitis, cystitis, or wound infection, for example, or those coming from tissue breakdown such as that following myocardial infarction, can prod the thermoregulatory center to produce hyperthermia, or fever. Cerebral edema, a cerebral vascular accident, neurosurgery, brain trauma, or tumor can also set the brain's thermostat at a higher level. The body responds by conserving and producing heat.

But hyperthermia may create hypoxia simply because the oxygen requirements of tissue metabolism increase 7% for every 1° F. rise in temperature. This means faster breathing and a rising pulse rate. The rapid breathing is to inhale more oxygen; the pulse shows that cardiac output has increased to try to meet the cellular need for that oxygen. But brain tissue is highly susceptible to hypoxia. Treatment is essential with cooling measures and O_2 if needed.

A slight fever is normal for a day or two after surgery. Otherwise, when a patient starts to run a fever, you should check all the daily intake and output records for the past several days. If the output is low and pushing fluids is not contraindicated (as it would be in congestive heart failure, cardiogenic shock, or increased intracranial pressure), you might increase the fluid intake for 2 hours while applying tepid sponges to the skin and perhaps lowering the room temperature. And if aspirin is ordered for the patient for other symptoms, you might give him one dose as an antipyretic. If the fever doesn't come down with these measures, notify the doctor.

The reason: Fever is the most common evidence of postoperative complications, usually pulmonary, wound or urinary infection, or thrombophlebitis. Pulmonary complications can often be prevented by chest physiotherapy, keeping an open airway, adequate hydration, and early ambulation. Head off wound infection by careful aseptic technique in dressing change. The most common cause of urinary infection is catheterization: Obviate it if you can by urging other voiding methods. Phlebitis can be discouraged if not prevented altogether by postop leg exercises, Ace bandages, and getting the patient around early.

In the beginning, the fever patient may have cool limbs; this means his superficial blood vessels are constricted to conserve

Probing the probes

The illustration on the opposite page shows the different kinds of thermometers currently in use: glass (centigrade and fahrenheit), disposable, and electronic. The probes for electronic thermometers serve different purposes. Those shown are: a general purpose probe for esophageal and rectal temperatures; a small flexible vinyl probe for esophageal temperatures in infants; a tubular probe for fast oral or rectal readings; an attachable surface probe for skin temperatures; a hypodermic probe in 18, 20, or 22 gauge for subcutaneous, intramuscular, intravenous, or small-area measurement; and a tissue implantation probe for long-term subcutaneous measurement.

heat, and his skin may appear pale or mottled. He may complain of feeling cold; he may shiver and shake with chills. A light blanket keeps him comfortable without increasing his temperature. But once the production of heat brings the body temperature up to the hypothalamic thermostat setting, he will no longer complain of cold. Then he will have frankly feverish signs.

When there is a sudden fever over 101° with chills, malaise, and growing confusion, faster, deeper breathing, faster pulse, and a sudden drop of systolic blood pressure below 80, look out for septic shock (see Chapter 14). Make sure of a clear airway and gas exchange, restore circulating blood volume, and notify the doctor, who will identify and treat the infection.

As a disease process stops, the hypothalamus setting returns to normal. Now the body's temperature is high enough for its own cooling mechanisms to be brought into play. General vasodilation reddens the skin and makes it hot to the touch. Intense sweating now cools the body by evaporation.

Hypothermia is sometimes medically induced to lower the oxygen requirements for surgical procedures such as heart or peripheral vascular surgery, neurosurgery, or amputation, and medical conditions such as gastrointestinal hemorrhage. Hypothermia can also be the result of accidental exposure. (General anesthesia for any surgery will produce something of the same effect: lowered metabolism, diminished circulation, pale, cool skin. So will shock.)

Take vital signs frequently for the hypothermic patient. Make sure he is attended constantly. Keep his airway open because his gag reflex may not be working. Turn him at least every 2 hours, and carry out passive range-of-motion. Observe the skin for discoloration or frostbite. In rewarming, take the same kind of care, and be sure he is not burned or overheated.

Pulse: The arterial wave

Each beat of the heart pumps blood into an already full aorta, flaring its walls and generating a fluid wave through the arteries: This wave is the pulse. The heart normally beats about 70 times a minute to send 5 liters of blood through the adult body. This cardiac output equals the volume of blood in each systole — the stroke volume — times the rate per minute: CO = SV x R. When the stroke volume lessens (as in shock), the rate increases, keeping the cardiac output constant. The rate is what you palpate at some peripheral artery as the pulse count.

To take the pulse, first inspect the patient and note any obvious pulsations. You can normally see pulsations in the neck of a recumbent patient, either as the brisk localized throbbing of the carotid artery, or the diffuse, undulant pulsation of the jugular vein. These pulsations ordinarily disappear as the patient is elevated to a sitting position, usually at 45°. When they do not, it can mean increased central venous pressure, as in heart failure. If this is a new sign, it should be reported. The doctor may want you to measure CVP (see Chapter 7).

Next, palpate the peripheral artery, using the pads of your first three fingers. Completely occlude the artery and release it gradually. For routine signs, the radial artery is usually the most accessible and can be easily compressed against the radius. In small children, the temporal artery is useful.

In the case of cardiac arrest, use a femoral or a carotid pulse to determine perfusion. But as a rule never put too much pressure on the carotid, lest that cause atrioventricular block, especially in patients who have had a myocardial infarction.

In the patient going to surgery, particularly for cardiac or peripheral vascular operations, assess all superficial pulses. Chart your baseline information for these:
- bilateral dorsalis pedis
- posterior tibialis
- popliteal
- femoral
- radial
- brachial

In this way nurses in the operating room, the recovery room, and the postop intensive care unit can determine if there are any postop changes.

All of these pulses should also be assessed in the medical patient entering the hospital for diabetes or for arterial occlusive conditions such as atherosclerosis, Raynaud's disease, Buerger's disease, and aneurysm. If a pulse is hard to palpate, mark its location with a felt pen so it'll be easier to find the next time. And if the peripheral pulse is abnormal in some way, you will also want to assess the apical heartbeat by auscultation.

You palpate the radial pulse not merely to determine its rate, but to assess the rhythm, force or amplitude, and quality, as well as elasticity.

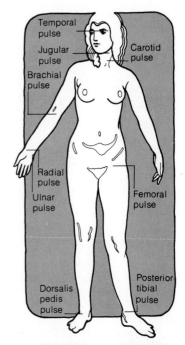

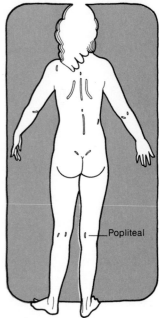

Pulse points

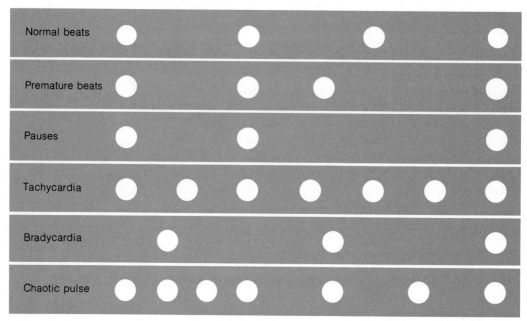

Normal beats	●	●	● ●
Premature beats	●	● ●	●
Pauses	●	●	●
Tachycardia	● ● ●	● ● ●	●
Bradycardia	●	●	●
Chaotic pulse	● ● ● ●	●	● ●

Watch the beat
This chart illustrates common irregularities in rate and rhythm that you will be able to feel when taking pulses.

Rate. Count the pulse for 30 seconds and multiply by two. But if you find any irregularities, then check it for at least a minute. For the resting adult, 60 to 100 beats a minute are normal, slightly faster in women than men, faster still in infants and children. There is also a mild increase in old age.

Tachycardia occurs with these conditions:
- pain
- anger, fear, anxiety
- exercise
- fever
- anemia
- hypoxia and CHF
- shock

Pain, as well as anger, fear, and anxiety all increase the heart rate by stimulating the sympathetic nervous system. Congestive heart failure, anemia, and fever all require greater oxygenation, therefore greater cardiac output. So does exercise: You must expect a patient's heart to beat faster if he has just been up.

Bradycardia comes with stimulation of the parasympathetic nervous system. This may commonly affect patients on digitalis, a drug that acts on the vagus nerves of the parasympathetic system. But bradycardia is also found in the fit athlete.

Rhythm should be regular, but there are two normal exceptions. Sinus arrhythmia, common in children and young adults, is an irregular pulse that speeds up at the peak of inspiration and slows down with expiration. Here's a test: When the patient holds his breath, the irregularity should disappear.

Another irregularity is an occasional premature beat. This occurs when some other pacemaker fires ahead of the sinoatrial node. Doing so prematurely, it initiates an early systole. Because of reduced filling time, the stroke volume is decreased enough for you to feel a pause in the rhythm. Almost everyone has the sensation occasionally of his heart "skipping a beat." But frequent premature ventricular contractions can indicate cardiac irritability, hypoxia, digitalis overdose, potassium imbalance — or they may be the danger sign of more serious arrhythmias. The patient may complain of palpitations or of feeling faint or dizzy.

If the patient's PVCs seem to come when he is in pain, an analgesic may be the solution. If the PVCs are due to hypoxia, then oxygen may help. The patient with myocardial infarction (who tolerates cardiac irritability poorly) may require a lidocaine drip or a bolus of some alternative antiarrhythmic drug. Depending upon what the synthesis of your present and previously collected data tells you, you may choose to limit visitors or reduce other stimuli such as noise. In other cases you may decide the physician should be notified.

Force or amplitude. The pulse pressure is the difference between systolic and diastolic pressure; amplitude is a reflection of pulse strength. When stroke volume increases with certain conditions such as anxiety, alcohol intake, or exercise, you can feel the pulse slap against your fingers, then collapse abruptly. This bounding pulse is also felt in pathological conditions such as complete heart block, anemia, hepatic failure, and the "water-hammer" (Corrigan's) pulse of aortic regurgitation.

Quality. The character of the pulse is usually noted on a three-point scale: 3+ is a bounding pulse, 2+ is normal, 1+ indicates a weak, thready pulse, and 0 an absent pulse.

Besides the bounding pulse and the bigeminal pulse (the one with the premature beat), you may also note paradoxical

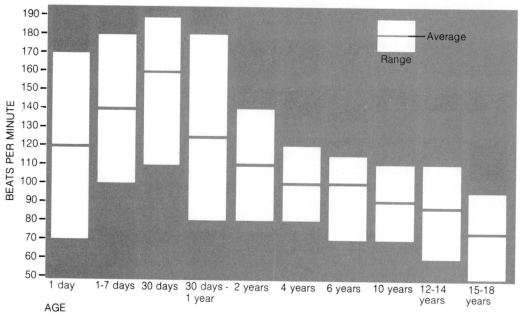

Range of rates
The chart above shows the normal range of pulse rates and average for children from birth to 18 years.

pulse. Like the sinus arrhythmia, this varies with breathing; here the force of the pulse is diminished when the patient inhales.

Both phenomena arise because inspiration traps more blood in the lungs and so decreases return to the left heart and consequent stroke volume. Paradoxical pulse is probably normal unless pronounced, when it may indicate cardiac tamponade. Other signs of the latter are dyspnea, high central venous pressure, distant and muffled heart sounds, narrowed pulse pressure, and falling blood pressure, as well as failing consciousness. This collection of blood or fluid in the pericardial sac is a medical emergency. Keep an aspirating needle and syringe ready, although the patient most likely will need surgery.

Elasticity is the expansibility or springiness of the normal arterial wall. It takes practice to assess this, but the flexible, non-tortuous artery of the normal patient feels very different from the hard, cord-like artery of atherosclerosis.

When you note any pulse irregularity, use the stethoscope to listen to the apical heartbeat, at the same time palpating the radial pulse to determine the pulse deficit, or difference between the two rates. Pass your findings to the physician.

Tutored practice is essential to auscultate heart sounds accurately (see Chapter 6).

Respiration: The ins and outs

The quality of normal relaxed breathing is effortless, automatic, regular and even, and almost silent. Start to assess it by inspection. While maintaining the patient's modesty, uncover the chest and inspect it. Does it expand symmetrically with inspiration? Is there any retraction of the interspaces on inspiration? If there is, suspect obstruction of the respiratory tract or the increased inspiratory effort of atelectasis. In children with respiratory obstruction or atelectasis, you will also note sternal retraction and nasal flaring. Bulging of a patient's interspaces, on the other hand, indicates trapped air, as in the forced expiration associated with asthma or emphysema.

The major muscle of normal breathing in both males and females is the diaphragm, though the chest wall in women may appear to move more than in men. But if the patient is using the intercostal muscles and the accessory muscles in the neck to help himself breathe, he may have chronic obstructive pulmonary disease in which he has difficulty getting the air out.

Be alert for dyspnea — difficult, labored breathing. The patient may even tell you he isn't getting enough air. His face looks anxious and tired from the exertion, nostrils flare with the increased inspiratory effort, and his color may be dusky. Still, charting that the patient is dyspneic does not tell much. Make a note of how much exertion it takes to produce the dyspnea: Is it from walking to the bathroom, or is he short of breath just from talking, pausing every few sentences to rest? Dyspnea also often goes with chronic obstructive pulmonary disease (COPD), or with left-sided heart failure.

Evaluate any sounds made by breathing. You will be able to hear bronchial sounds over the large airways. These are fairly loud and of a high pitch. Exhalation is slower than inspiration, with a slight pause between them. Softer, lower vesicular sounds will be heard over the other lung areas and have no pause between inspiration and exhalation. Any noisy breathing is obstructed breathing. If the breathing is noisy, you may elect to suction the patient or, unless there are contraindications, to increase his activity. Or, you may decide he needs coughing and deep-breathing exercises. If the patient is not fully conscious, he may require an oral or nasal airway.

How to describe breath sounds

Respiratory sounds have their own list of names. Here are some:

Stertorous — snoring sound due to secretions in the trachea and large bronchi. Watch for this in neurologic or comatose patients.

Stridor — the inspiratory crowing sound that occurs with upper airway obstruction in laryngitis, the lodging of a foreign body, or croup in children.

Wheeze — the high-pitched, musical sound that occurs with partial obstruction in the smaller bronchi and bronchioles, as in emphysema or asthma.

Sigh — a very deep inspiration followed by a prolonged expiration. Occasional sighs are normal and purposeful, to expand alveoli. Frequent sighs may indicate emotional tension.

Rales and *rhonchi* — rattling sounds that occur with secretions in the lung passageways. To categorize these breath sounds accurately, a stethoscope and tutored practice are necessary (see Chapter 4).

Expiratory grunt — in infants this indicates imminent respiratory distress; in older patients, it may be caused by a partial airway obstruction or a neuromuscular reflex.

Absence of sound — a result of any condition, such as pneumothorax, atelectasis, or local airway obstruction, that prevents the ventilation of part or all of a lung field.

Besides the quality of respirations, you will want to notice their rate, depth, and pattern. Rate and depth make up the type of respiration. The normal rate at rest is 12-18 breaths per minute in adults, 24-34 in infants about 2 years old, and 20-26 in children about 10 years old. The ratio of pulse to respirations is fairly constant, about 5:1. Count the respiratory rate for at least 30 seconds, and for a full minute if you suspect any abnormality. Counting for only 15 seconds can give a misleading count of +4, which is significant when working with such small numbers. Sometimes you might have to wait for a second count: People suddenly conscious of their breathing tend to alter it involuntarily.

The depth is the volume of air moving in and out with each respiration. This tidal volume is normally about 500 cc in the adult and should be constant with each breath. To measure the amount precisely, you need a portable spirometer such as the Wright Respirometer. But you can tell whether the depth is adequate by placing the back of your hand close to the nose and mouth and feeling the exhaled air, while observing whether there is adequate and symmetrical chest expansion.

The lungs' function is to maintain homeostasis of arterial blood. By retaining or venting carbon dioxide, respiration, helped by the kidneys, maintains the pH of the blood. When there is metabolic acidosis, the rate and depth of breathing become much greater. This is a compensation that serves to blow off CO_2 and, so, neutralize the excess amounts of hydrogen ions, the basis of the acidemia. Conversely, if there is metabolic alkalosis, the body attempts, though less effectively, to compensate by retaining the CO_2. In severe metabolic alkalosis, the rate of breathing is decreased, the depth is shallow, and the respiratory pattern is disrupted by periods of apnea lasting from 5 to 30 seconds.

Besides the quality, type, and pattern of the patient's respiration, you should also record any significant physical characteristics. Persons with COPD, for example, have an anterior-posterior chest diameter as big as their transverse one because of the chronic overinflation of the lungs. Their ribs flare horizontally instead of sloping downward. Very often they sit leaning forward with their arms braced against their knees, a chair, or the bed to compress the abdomen and increase intrathoracic pressure.

Whatever their primary ailment, patients with asthma, em-

How to describe changes in respiratory rate

Use the following terms only if everyone on your floor is familiar with them. If not, describe the specific character.

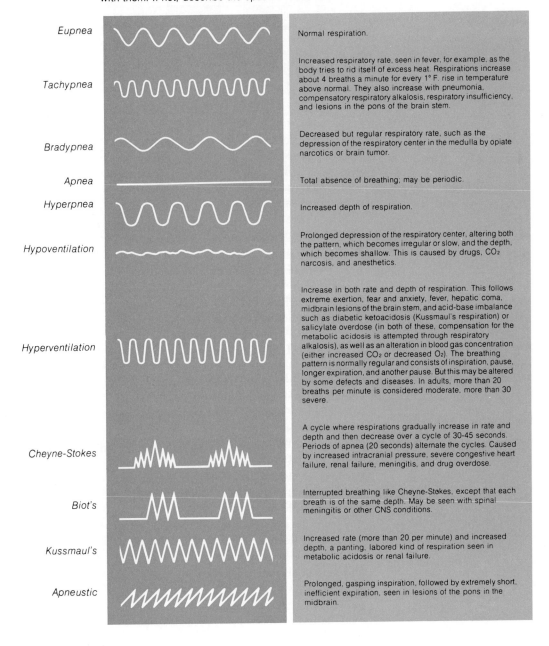

Eupnea — Normal respiration.

Tachypnea — Increased respiratory rate, seen in fever, for example, as the body tries to rid itself of excess heat. Respirations increase about 4 breaths a minute for every 1° F. rise in temperature above normal. They also increase with pneumonia, compensatory respiratory alkalosis, respiratory insufficiency, and lesions in the pons of the brain stem.

Bradypnea — Decreased but regular respiratory rate, such as the depression of the respiratory center in the medulla by opiate narcotics or brain tumor.

Apnea — Total absence of breathing; may be periodic.

Hyperpnea — Increased depth of respiration.

Hypoventilation — Prolonged depression of the respiratory center, altering both the pattern, which becomes irregular or slow, and the depth, which becomes shallow. This is caused by drugs, CO_2 narcosis, and anesthetics.

Hyperventilation — Increase in both rate and depth of respiration. This follows extreme exertion, fear and anxiety, fever, hepatic coma, midbrain lesions of the brain stem, and acid-base imbalance such as diabetic ketoacidosis (Kussmaul's respiration) or salicylate overdose (in both of these, compensation for the metabolic acidosis is attempted through respiratory alkalosis), as well as an alteration in blood gas concentration (either increased CO_2 or decreased O_2). The breathing pattern is normally regular and consists of inspiration, pause, longer expiration, and another pause. But this may be altered by some defects and diseases. In adults, more than 20 breaths per minute is considered moderate, more than 30 severe.

Cheyne-Stokes — A cycle where respirations gradually increase in rate and depth and then decrease over a cycle of 30-45 seconds. Periods of apnea (20 seconds) alternate the cycles. Caused by increased intracranial pressure, severe congestive heart failure, renal failure, meningitis, and drug overdose.

Biot's — Interrupted breathing like Cheyne-Stokes, except that each breath is of the same depth. May be seen with spinal meningitis or other CNS conditions.

Kussmaul's — Increased rate (more than 20 per minute) and increased depth, a panting, labored kind of respiration seen in metabolic acidosis or renal failure.

Apneustic — Prolonged, gasping inspiration, followed by extremely short, inefficient expiration, seen in lesions of the pons in the midbrain.

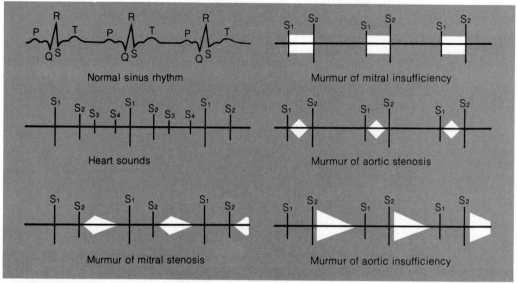

Normal sinus rhythm

Murmur of mitral insufficiency

Heart sounds

Murmur of aortic stenosis

Murmur of mitral stenosis

Murmur of aortic insufficiency

Sick at heart
Using the chart above, you can compare the various sounds of the heart. An EKG represents graphically the electrical activity of the heart whereas the vibrations of the heart produce the sounds you hear with auscultation. In mitral stenosis you will hear a low-pitched rumbling murmur during ventricular diastole.

When the mitral valve is insufficient, you will hear a high-pitched blowing murmur on systole. Aortic stenosis produces a medium-pitched, harsh sound during systole. And aortic insufficiency produces a high-pitched, blowing murmur during diastole.

physema, chronic bronchitis, or all three are surely going to need pulmonary hygiene at regular intervals, low-flow oxygen in periods of distress, and retraining in breathing so that they learn to expel the back-up air. Pursed-lip breathing is one of the most valuable exercises for this.

Note down any chest deformity — scoliosis, funnel chest, pigeon breast. These, too, could interfere with breathing. Look at the skin for pallor or cyanosis, especially of sudden onset. Cyanosis is the bluish color coming from an increased amount of reduced hemoglobin in the superficial blood vessels. The best place to look for it is under the tongue or on the buccal mucosa (see Chapter 2 for a fuller explanation). Remember that peripheral blood flow can be unrelated to the adequacy of respiration — though it can be a weather vane for the onset of heart failure or shock. (Remember also, in patients with any obstructive chest disease, cyanosis may be a late sign and so of little diagnostic value.)

Why is the sudden onset of cyanosis ordinarily so important to notice? Because it indicates hypoxia. With it, look for restlessness, irritability, confusion, impaired motor function, and heightened pulse, respiration, and blood pressure. Give oxygen for this set of signs. If the hypoxia is prolonged, the patient may become diaphoretic and lose consciousness, and eventually the blood pressure will collapse.

Blood pressure: The dynamics of circulation

Blood flows from heart to artery to capillary to vein by differences in their internal pressure, pressure being least in the veins. These vascular pressures are controlled by the vasomotor center in the medulla oblongata. This center signals for constriction or expansion of the muscular walls of the vessels. This alters pressure and, so, circulation by shrinking or enlarging the container. Mostly the difference is temporary. Sometimes, by reason of physiologic change, it lasts.

That means, blood pressure varies not only with the moment but with condition. It is lowest in neonates and climbs with age, as it does with weight gain, continued stress, or anxiety. Most likely to develop hypertension are people living in urban environments, those subjected to emotional distress, U.S. blacks, and women (2 to 1 over men). Exercise drives blood pressure up temporarily, as does pain or rage. So, for a longer time, do several disease states.

Shock, myocardial infarction, and hemorrhage are among the things that drop it, because they reduce cardiac output or peripheral vessel resistance, or they lessen venous return after fluid loss. (But even in shock, excitement may hold the blood pressure high or normal, at least for a while.)

By its own hemodynamics, then, you can expect the blood pressure to be an index to:

- elasticity of the arterial walls
- peripheral vascular resistance
- efficiency of the heart as a pump
- blood volume

When you take a blood pressure reading, you measure the systolic pressure, the diastolic pressure and, by subtraction, the pulse pressure, the difference between them. A reasonable systolic pressure — the maximum exertion against the arteries by the left ventricular systole — is a clue to the integrity of heart, arteries, and arterioles. The diastolic pressure, constantly present on the arterial walls, directly indicates blood vessel resistance. The pulse pressure tends to parallel the cardiac stroke volume.

But remember just the same, a single blood pressure reading is almost always inaccurate. You must know the average vital signs for your patient before you attach significance to one isolated figure.

The average blood pressure in a young adult (but often

How to get the right blood pressure reading

To avoid falsely high or low readings in taking blood pressure, know how to eliminate the errors than can produce them. Here are errors that give a falsely *elevated* B/P:

• using too narrow a cuff: The cuff bladder should be 20% wider than the diameter of the extremity in use. Remember this in taking a thigh pressure or even the pressure of an obese person.
• wrapping the cuff too loosely.
• deflating the cuff too slowly; venous congestion in the extremity will give a false high.
• tilting the mercury column away from the vertical.
• having the mercury column above eye level.
• taking a reading in a patient who is upset or has just eaten or ambulated.

Errors producing a falsely *low* B/P:

• having a patient's arm above the level of his heart.
• having the mercury column below eye level.
• failure to notice an "auscultatory gap"; in this instance, the sound, after fading out for 10-15 mm Hg, returns. But if you do not pump the cuff high enough, you will miss the top sound. To avoid this, palpate the radial artery as you pump the cuff.
• inability to hear feeble sounds. If you cannot hear them, have the patient raise his arm before you inflate the cuff again. This decreases venous pressure and should make the sounds louder. Then lower the arm, deflate the cuff, and listen. If you still cannot hear, chart the palpatory systolic pressure.

variable at that) is 120/80 mm Hg. The World Health Organization defines hypertension as a persistent elevation above 140/90; hypotension in adults is often given as below 95/60. Even so, hypotension in the healthy adult, shown as a persistent systolic pressure of 90 to 100 but without accompanying symptoms, is no cause for alarm.

Everybody's blood pressure is usually lowest in the early morning after sleep. It rises after meals, during exercise, or with emotional upset. It's lower when a patient is lying down than when he's sitting or standing. And it's a little higher in the lower extremities. But whether you are going to take a sitting or supine reading, keep the patient in a stable, relaxed position for 5-10 minutes, and be sure he hasn't eaten or exercised for 30. Also be sure his arm is at heart level.

Taking the pressure. Put the center of the cuff over the brachial artery, and wrap the cuff evenly. Palpate the radial artery, inflate the cuff as rapidly as possible until the pulse you are feeling is gone, and then pump for an extra 20-30 mm Hg beyond that.

Place the diaphragm of your stethoscope over the brachial artery and release the cuff at a rate of 2 mm Hg per heartbeat. The systolic pressure is the reading at the first return of the sound.

As the cuff is released, you'll hear a damping or muffling of the sound. The American Heart Association accepts this as the most accurate index of diastolic pressure, but recommends recording both that and the final distinct sound as the complete record, so: 120/80/78.

Some clinicians say that a 10 to 20 mm Hg gain or drop — with no history of such flexibility and no change in exercise level or bed position — should be investigated. Then you have to rule out other variables: For example, has the patient's respiratory status changed, requiring more work to breathe? Or has the I.V. changed its rate, say, because the patient moved from his side to his back, causing an alteration in circulatory load?

Hypertension comes with such factors as kidney disease, coarctation of the aorta, viscous blood (such as that in polycythemia), or endocrine disorders, among them pheochromocytoma, an adrenal tumor causing headache, blurred vision, sweating, palpitations, and rapid heartbeat. There is also essential hypertension of no known cause. There is a strong familial tendency for hypertension, and the patient may have nosebleeds and severe headaches as well and show irritability.

Also classified as hypertension are conditions where the systolic pressure is increased even though the diastolic remains normal. These may include anemia, hyperthyroidism, aortic insufficiency, and, in an older patient, atherosclerosis.

In the neurosurgical patient or the one with brain trauma, elevated blood pressure or a widened pulse pressure with a low pulse rate may also be a danger sign meaning increased intracranial pressure. Watch him closely for clouding of consciousness, changes in movement (hemiparesis, positive Babinski reflex), or inequality of pupil sizes. Notify the doctor of these changes at once. A late sign may be Cheyne-Stokes respiration. If you see any of these changes in such a patient, take his vital signs every 15 minutes until they are stable.

Hypertension both comes from and worsens kidney disease. In such cases, keep alert also for severe headache, blurred vision, marked loss of weight, and signs of renal failure. In helping the patient, the blood pressure must be controlled.

Coarctation (congenital narrowing) of the aorta, usually found in the teenager or young adult, often shows a surprisingly high blood pressure in both arms, with pressure in the legs — normally higher — much lower because the blood supply to the legs is below the constriction.

Hypotension occurs when the total blood volume is decreased, as it is in shock from hemorrhage, burns, vomiting, diarrhea, metabolic acidosis, heat exhaustion, or Addisonian crisis. (One of the earliest signs of hypovolemia is a decreased urine volume.) Hypotension also occurs with decreased cardiac output, such as an acute myocardial infarction.

Hypotension is not always easy to define: A normally hypertensive patient may actually be hypotensive at 150/90. Watch here for change and for other signs and symptoms. You can expect a small drop in the blood pressure, for example, when you apply blankets to warm up a postop patient who is vasoconstricted from the cool operating room. If the drop is not significant, and the pulse remains stable, you can assume that the adjustment is normal. But if the drop continues, the pulse increases, and the patient starts to perspire, inspect him for signs of hemorrhage. Notify the doctor of the change.

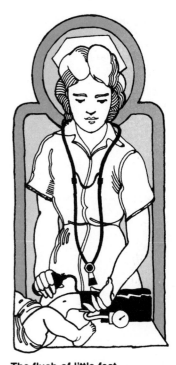

The flush of little feet
To avoid the difficulties of obtaining precise blood pressure readings on neonates, you can use the flush method, which shows the mean diastolic-systolic pressure. Using a sphygmomanometer, wrap a neonatal cuff just above the ankle (you can also use the wrist). Squeeze the extremity below the cuff as you pump the manometer to 120-140 mm Hg. This will blanch the baby's leg below the cuff. Next, release your hand as you release the gauge at a rate of no more than 5 mm Hg per second. Record the Hg level at which you notice the baby's leg flush. That is the mean diastolic-systolic pressure.

The hypotension of shock or myocardial infarction is accompanied not only by an increased pulse rate and heavy sweating, but also dizziness, confusion, and blurred vision. The skin feels cool and clammy as vasoconstriction begins to shunt blood to the vital organs. Treatment depends on the type of shock, as Chapters 13 and 14 suggest. But in all cases, assess vital signs and mental status frequently. You'll also need venous blood for chemistries; this can be drawn when the I.V. is started.

The patient who has a myocardial infarction in addition to the above signs may also complain of crushing substernal pain, high epigastric pain, or arm, shoulder, or jaw pain. He needs morphine for the pain (give it I.V. so it will not alter his enzyme results), oxygen, complete rest, and I.V. fluids. Raising the leg gatch (with no knee break) may overcome the hypotension. Start as many of these measures as you can manage before he is transferred to ICU.

Another alteration in blood pressure is paradoxical blood pressure. The sound of it varies with the patient's breathing, fading out with inspiration and becoming stronger with expiration — much like paradoxical pulse. This is a perfectly normal occurrence with very deep breathing. But if it occurs for no seeming reason, or is pronounced, it may mean cardiac tamponade.

With experience, you'll add observations of your own to these necessarily brief descriptions. But essentially, making the most of vital signs means to:
- take them at the right times, as often as needed
- see how they have changed from previous values
- determine how they fit into the patient's entire clinical picture
- take whatever nursing measures you feel are needed, and check the signs again.

If you decide the doctor must be notified, give him all the information you have been able to gather about these bodily indicators.

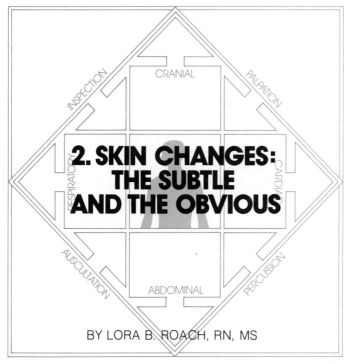

2. SKIN CHANGES: THE SUBTLE AND THE OBVIOUS

BY LORA B. ROACH, RN, MS

WHILE YOU IMMEDIATELY THINK of vital signs in patient assessment, you also must remember that the skin mirrors disease. So, you must know how to see the reflection clearly — how to detect changes in skin condition…distinguish between simple erythema and a macular rash…recognize early cyanosis or jaundice.

As obvious as skin conditions would seem to be, though, they aren't always easy to detect. Remember that people tend to consider skin lesions as disfiguring and shameful. So, many may deliberately conceal a lesion or abnormality with jewelry, clothing, cosmetics or professional cover-up preparations. While examining skin, listen carefully to the patient's comments and answers to your questions. Sometimes an evasive answer will hint at concealed lesions.

Remember, too, that concealment can occur naturally — as in darkly pigmented skin. The normal distribution patterns of pigment in dark-skinned persons may obscure certain color changes, and lead to misinterpretations by inexperienced observers. For example, some dark-skinned people, particularly of Mediterranean origin, have very blue lips, giving a false impression of cyanosis. Full-blooded blacks often have normal bluish pigmentation of the gums, distributed evenly or in splotches; the portion of the sclera exposed in the lid slit may contain deposits of brown melanin that could be misinterpreted as petechiae. Also, blacks commonly have brown, freckle-like pigmentation of the gums, buccal cavity, borders of the tongue, and even of the nail beds. Babies of genetically dark-skinned persons are lightly pigmented at birth, but grow progressively darker with age until pigmentation peaks after six to eight weeks. You can best observe color changes in both the adult and child where pigmentation from melanin, melanoid and carotene is least: the sclera, conjunctiva, nail beds, lips, buccal mucosa, tongue, palms and soles. However, heavily calloused palms and soles usually have an opaque yellowish cast (carotene), which decreases their value to the observer.

Finally, remember that lipstick, nail polish, hair dye, and wigs may inadvertently obscure changes or lesions. Certain occupations or children's play can cause coverings of sweat, dust, or grease, which hinder satisfactory examination. When cleansing is indicated, take care not to create additional injury or distortion of color through use of vigorous friction or harsh soaps.

Getting the right light
Inadequate lighting often hampers observation of color changes such as pallor, cyanosis, and jaundice. Some fluorescent lights cause even healthy people to appear cyanotic. The best illumination is non-glare daylight but, in its absence, one of the new lights that simulate sunlight may be satisfactory. If this is not available, use a stand light with a bulb of at least 60 watts. Do not use a flashlight or the soft illumination of most overbed lights. They are totally inadequate for identifying subtle color changes.

When examining the skin, remember to consider and control, when possible, the influencing forces of gravity, environmental temperature, emotions, and cigarette smoking. Chilling, anger, fright, and cigarette smoking — all cause varying degrees of peripheral vasoconstriction and hide pallor and cyanosis. Excessive warmth and embarrassment can cause an increased redness that mimics erythema and masks many signs of pathology.

Remember, too, the relationship between bodily position

and vascular function. The skin of a leg may look as if it has a satisfactory blood supply while the patient is in bed with his leg at heart level. When he sits with his leg dependent, however, it may become cyanotic, demonstrating impaired vascular integrity. Here's a good method to assess a relationship between coloration and the position of an extremity: Examine the part while it is at heart level, then (assuming there are no contra-indications), elevate the part about 15 degrees for at least 5 minutes, and finally lower it 30 to 90 degrees for at least 5 minutes.

Using the best examining methods

During inspection of the skin and mucous membrane, look for changes or abnormalities of color, contour, integrity, and hygiene. Also, be alert for behavior that suggests skin disorders, such as scratching, rubbing, and picking the skin.

During palpation, evaluate texture, temperature, and secretions of the skin and its appendages. Evaluate sensitivity to touch and localized temperature.

Smell is a technique of observation that is not well developed in most nurses, because humans are not noted for their ability to discriminate between differing odors. The skin, as well as the breath, often has an odor. The skin of uremia patients, for example, will often have an odor of urine.

Use all three of these observational methods concurrently, skillfully, and with good interview techniques, and you will increase the accuracy of your nursing diagnoses.

Starting with specific observations

Observation of color tells you something about the patient's vascular function and his nutritional status. It can also reveal certain poisonings. Inspect for abnormal colors, increase or decrease of the natural color, distribution of color, luster (whether translucent or opaque), and other qualities (brilliant, dull, "dirty").

You can best observe slight color changes of pallor, cyanosis, and jaundice where capillary beds are superficial and pigmentation is minimal — the conjunctiva, nail beds, lips, hard palate, and palms and soles.

Pinpointing pallor and its causes

Pallor may stem from a person's natural coloring. If so, the

What the nose knows

If you learn to use odors as a diagnostic tool, your olfactory sense will help you identify many infections and diseases. Below a helpful checklist shows you what conditions certain smells may presage.

new-mown clover — hepatic failure
sweet fruity odor — diabetic acidosis
paraldehyde — acute poisoning
bitter almond — cyanide poisoning
garlic — arsenic poisoning
burnt rope — marijuana
camphor — ingestion of mothballs (pica)
stale urine — uremic acidosis
overripe cheese — isovaleric acidemia
musty or horsey odor — phenylketonuria
halitosis — gingival inflammation or stomatitis
nasal malodor — chronic postnasal drip, pharyngitis, or rhinitis.

skin should look healthy and translucent, and the mucous membranes and nail beds should be pink. Anemia usually causes a sallow skin (pale, sickly, yellowish) and pale mucous membranes. Acute blood loss makes the mucous membranes almost white and the skin very white, waxy looking, cool, and moist.

Evaluate degree of pallor by inspecting the color of the patient's palms while he is lying down, hands at heart level. (Blood flow to the hand increases considerably in the supine position.) The palms demonstrate pallor early because of decreased hemoglobin in the blood, and the creases in the palm become pale in cases of severe anemia.

When you suspect pallor caused by internal hemorrhage or a cardiovascular dysfunction (including a localized obstruction such as a tight arm cast), do a capillary-filling test. Apply a slight pressure on the free edge of the patient's second or third fingernail, blanching the nail bed. Then note the speed with which the color returns after you slowly release the pressure. A slow return, as compared with a test of your own nails, indicates diminished quality of vasomotor function. You can test other tissues, particularly the lips and ear lobes, in much the same way if the patient's nails are unusable for the test. These tests work as well with dark-skinned patients as with light-skinned patients.

Seeing cyanosis

Essentially the same technique is used to detect cyanosis as for pallor. The nail beds readily demonstrate cyanosis. But do not be misled by "cold cyanosis" caused in sensitive individuals by an uncomfortably low environmental temperature. The palpebral conjunctiva demonstrates generalized cyanosis as readily as it does pallor. But you need to become thoroughly familiar with the pre-cyanotic color to recognize early changes. Usually cyanosis can best be seen in the skin around the lips, the cheeks, and ear lobes because these tissues are thick and highly vascular.

Cyanosis remains the most difficult clinical sign to observe in the darkly pigmented individual. The usual sites of observation may have just enough pigmentation to obscure beginning cyanosis. Nevertheless, close inspection of the lips, nail beds, palpebral conjunctiva, palms, and soles at regular intervals will usually enable you to recognize cyanosis when it de-

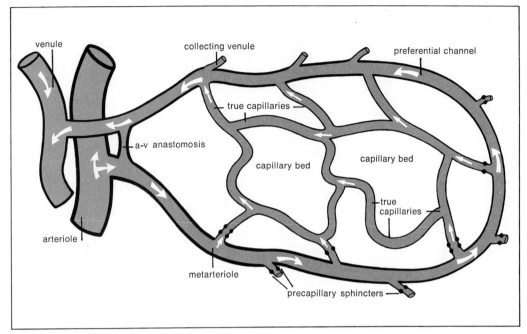

velops. Follow the same procedures you would in a light-pigmented individual.

You may need to differentiate between cardiovascular-related cyanosis and other causes of bluish-gray color, such as the presence of methemoglobin and deposits of silver or bismuth. To do that, perform the capillary-filling test directly on the cyanotic skin (or nail bed). Apply light pressure to create pallor. In cyanosis, the color returns slowly by spreading from the periphery to the center. Normally, the color returns in less than one second and it appears to return from below the pallid spot as well as from the periphery. If chemical deposits are present, the bluish-gray color remains evident in the pallid spot and may even obscure the characteristics of capillary filling, which would be normal if discernible.

Distribution of cyanosis is particularly important in your assessment. For example, peripheral cyanosis of the hands, feet, and tip of the nose is particularly characteristic of low-output cardiac failure, whereas central or generalized cyanosis is characteristic of impaired gas exchange between the alveoli and the pulmonary capillaries. To differentiate between central and peripheral cyanosis, massage a small portion of the

Feeling blue?
Central cyanosis, shown above, is characterized by a normal flow of blood that does not, however, carry sufficient oxygen to nourish the cells. In peripheral cyanosis the blood may contain enough oxygen but the blood flow itself is inadequate.

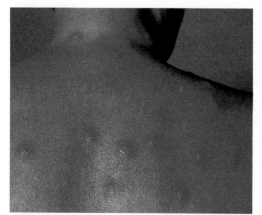

Drug reaction: tetanus toxin

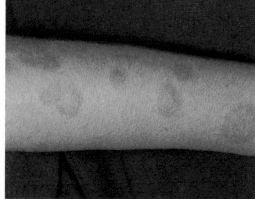

Drug reaction (fixed): barbiturates

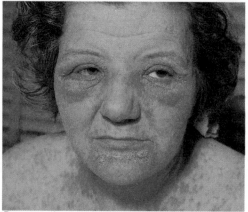

Drug reaction: penicillin

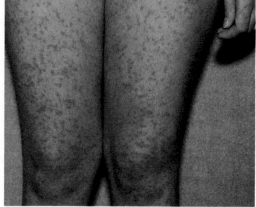

Drug reaction: ampicillin

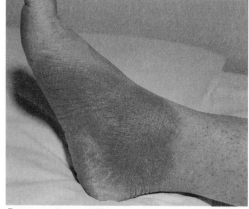

Drug reaction: aspirin

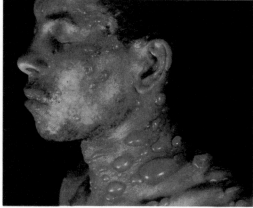

Drug reaction (bulbous): sulfathiazole

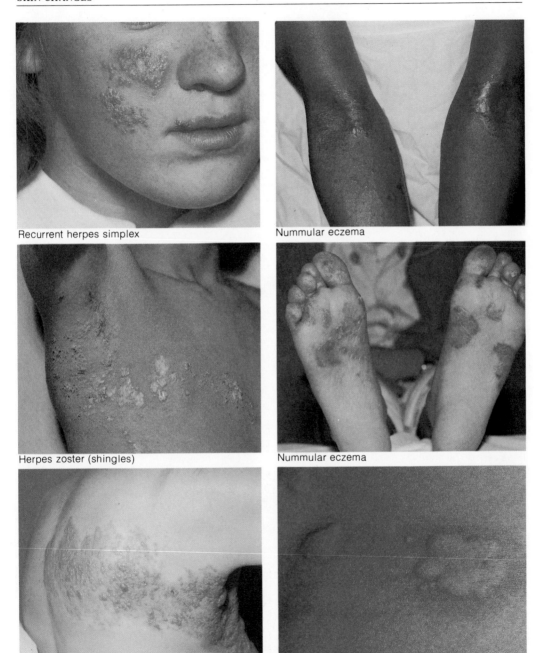

Recurrent herpes simplex

Nummular eczema

Herpes zoster (shingles)

Nummular eczema

Herpes zoster

Chronic urticaria (hives)

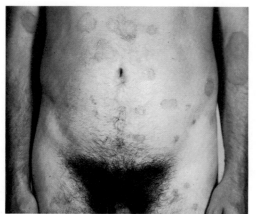

Tinea (ringworm) corporis

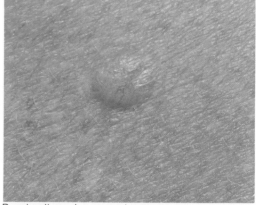

Basal cell carcinoma: early stage

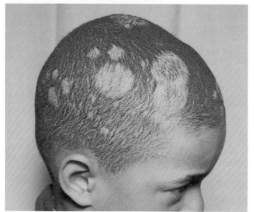

Tinea capitis

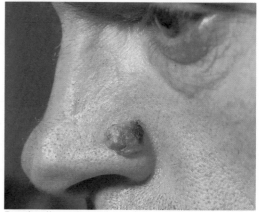

Basal cell carcinoma

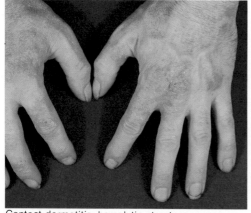

Contact dermatitis: hemolytic streptococcus

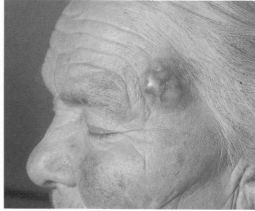

Basal cell carcinoma

cyanotic skin. If the cyanosis is peripheral, it will disappear upon massage; if central, it will not. Peripheral vasoconstriction — as caused by generalized chilling, smoking, and medications — can displace or prevent cyanosis even though serious anoxia is present.

Remember to control influencing factors such as smoking and excessive air-conditioning throughout the observation period. Peripheral vasoconstriction can prevent cyanosis even though serious anoxia is present. Also, for cyanosis to be evident, the blood must contain 5 grams of reduced hemoglobin or 1.5 grams of methemoglobin per 100 ml of blood.

Erythema and its complications

Erythema presents more problems in observation than pallor and cyanosis do. Simple inspection will readily reveal either a local or a generalized increase in redness. Such information, however, is too incomplete. You must also observe color tone, quality, distribution, and related factors. For example, is the increased color distributed over the face, neck, and thorax; is it a bright, cherry red flush? If so, suspect acute carbon monoxide poisoning. Is there redness of the palms? If so, suspect cirrhosis of the liver. Or is the diffuse red rash distributed symmetrically over the trunk and thighs? Then suspect drug sensitivity. Is the erythema accompanied by increased skin temperature? If so, look for fever or inflammation. Is it associated with lesions or itching?

When you suspect inflammation, palpate for increased warmth, for slick, tight skin suggesting edema, and for hardening of deep tissues or blood vessels. (With dark-skinned patients, this technique may provide your only clue to inflammation.) The dorsal surface of your fingers will be more sensitive to subtle temperature differences than will the palmar surface. Curve your fingers into a relaxed flexion and gently rest the middle phalanges on the skin to be tested; then move them to another skin surface for comparison.

The erythema of rash is not always accompanied by a noticeable increase in skin temperature. With a little practice in palpating different skin textures, you can usually identify papular rash by palpating gently with the fingertips. In the case of macular rash concealed by heavy pigmentation, you may have to rely on the patient's complaints of itching, or on evidence of scratching. Keep in mind, though, that itching may result from a number of other conditions such as jaundice, dry skin, irritating clothing or chemicals.

If you have difficulty distinguishing between a macular rash and simple erythema, stretch the skin gently between your thumb and finger (as for administering an injection). This maneuver decreases the red tone of erythema but accentuates macules. You can use the same maneuver to help differentiate petechiae and ecchymoses from erythema.

Looking for hemorrhagic lesions

In liver disease, venules on the trunk, face, and arms become distended, and spider angiomas (small, bright red, pulsating arterioles that disappear with pressure) frequently appear. Small areas of hemorrhage or petechiae appear in people with thrombocytopenia or liver disease. In people predisposed to these conditions, inspect the conjunctiva, buccal mucosa, and the skin over bony prominences (especially of dependent areas). Also examine the patient's arm carefully before and after you take the arterial blood pressure. The tourniquet effect of the inflated cuff increases the intracapillary pressure, which could cause rupture if there is peripheral vascular disease.

You can see larger hemorrhagic lesions (ecchymoses and hematomas) easily if they aren't covered by clothing. Color changes that occur with time (from reddish-purple to blue-black, to greenish-brown, to yellow) provide useful information about the probable age of the lesion. Always obtain as much information as possible about the history of any lesion to distinguish between spontaneous bleeding and that induced by trauma.

Judging jaundice

Detecting jaundice, a distinctive sign of liver malfunction, is somewhat complicated by the possibility of other causes of yellow color, including a fading suntan, excessive carotene, cholesterol, drugs (quinacrine, picric acid), and industrial chemicals. You can differentiate by inspecting the patient's sclera and hard palate. Yellowish fatty deposits in the sclera become heavier as the distance from the cornea increases. So, inspecting the portion of the sclera revealed naturally by the lid slit may provide the most accurate assessment of color, particularly in dark-skinned patients. When the sclera looks yellow even to the edges of the cornea, inspect the posterior portion of the hard palate in bright daylight. Jaundice can be detected there quite early, when serum bilirubin is 2 to 4 mg per 100 ml. The absence of a yellowish tint of the palate when the sclerae are yellow would indicate carotene pigmentation rather than jaundice. None of the other producers of yellow coloring will localize to any extent in the sclera and palate except picric acid; a history of its ingestion will usually differentiate it from jaundice.

Scratch marks provide contributory but not definite information. Itching is present in about only one-fourth of people with jaundice and may accompany many other disorders as well.

Don't wait until the skin is yellow to examine the sclera for jaundice. If edema precedes jaundice, the skin will not become yellow until very late. Edema of the skin reduces the intensity of skin color by increasing the distance between the surface and the pigmented and vascular layers.

Knowing why melanin varies

Changes in the number and distribution of melanin deposits often occur with hormonal and neurologic disorders. Melanization may increase so gradually that it goes unnoticed or is attributed to suntanning. Look for melanization of the sclera and buccal mucosa, too. Distributive patterns of melanin (and absence of melanin) are, as a rule, not distinctive for specific diseases. But when combined with other findings such as texture and contour, they may provide diagnostic evidence. Patients with connective tissue diseases: scleroderma (or dermatomyositis), thyrotoxicosis, chronic tuberculosis, or Addison's disease tend to have an increase in melanization.

Feeling texture and contour

Examining texture and contour requires practice to train your fingertips to recognize differences. A light, stroking movement will distinguish surface quality and contour of the skin (smooth, dry, scaly, papular). Stroking will also detect deposits (urate crystals, salt). A gentle pressing and pinching movement helps gauge elasticity and thickness of the skin, and quality of the subcutaneous tissue (waxy, doughy, flabby). Test skin turgor by pinching and releasing the skin of the patient's inner forearm. Normally, it returns to its original

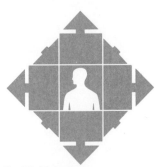

Health history:
What you should know
1. Does the patient have a history of dermatological problems? When was the onset? Any recurrence? What was the site, the nature of any lesions? Were there any additional signs and symptoms? What treatment was used? With what results?
2. Does he have any problems now? Does he suffer any related pain? Does he have allergies? What medications does he take? Does he use cosmetics?
3. Is his condition the result of or aggravated by his habits of sleep, hygiene, or diet?

shape almost immediately, but with excess sodium loss, the skin remains folded for 30 seconds or longer. Advanced age and severe malnutrition (cachexia) decrease skin turgor without sodium loss.

Identifying edema

You can sometimes detect edema by inspecting, but you need to palpate to identify the type and classify it on a scale of +1 to 4, the most severe. Location of edematous fluid is determined by the force of gravity, so examine the most dependent tissues (feet and ankles of ambulatory patients; presacral and pretibial tissue of bedfast patients). Press firmly into the tissue with your thumb for 5-10 seconds. A depression that does not promptly return to the normal contour indicates pitting edema. When testing other sites, always apply pressure over a bony surface.

You can identify non-pitting edema by using firm pressing and feeling motions of the fingers and thumb to detect the tight skin and subcutaneous hardness of edematous tissue. Unless inflammation accompanies the edema, the skin will usually feel slightly cool. Not all localized swelling is edema, so palpate carefully for the more compressible, fluctuant feel of a pocket of fluid, or the crackling feel (crepitation) of subcutaneous emphysema (air).

Testing integrity

To assess disruptions of integrity of skin and mucous membrane, use inspection, palpation, and smell. Some types of lesions defy assessment because of drainage, debris, and scratch marks. So, look for the original or basic lesion, and note its characteristics (papular, vesicular, pustular, open, closed, trauma-induced) and the condition of the adjacent tissue (clean, dirty, pallid, erythematous, edematous, cyanotic). When the lesions are still intact, palpate for skin temperature and tenderness or pain. Palpation not only yields information, but it may also benefit the patient. Touch is an important way to communicate affection and concern, and in the presence of disfiguring lesions, it may help negate the patient's feelings of degradation.

Making other observations

Note the odor of all lesions. Some have no detectable odor, but

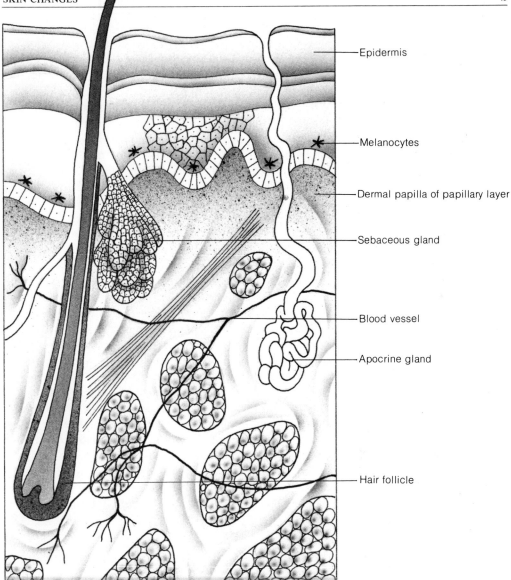

Epidermis

Melanocytes

Dermal papilla of papillary layer

Sebaceous gland

Blood vessel

Apocrine gland

Hair follicle

Skin deep

Melanocytes, the cells that produce the pigment melanin, are located at the junction of the epidermis and dermis. Light penetrates the superficial strata of the skin and is reflected by the underlying pigment, giving skin a normally translucent appearance. Melanin provides shades of yellow, brown, and black to the skin; melanoid and carotene provide additional tints of yellow. The superficial capillaries and venous plexuses allow the color of oxyhemoglobin (red) and reduced hemoglobin (blue) to shine through the epidermis, giving the skin various shades of color. Rapid changes in red or blue are caused by variations in the caliber of superficial blood vessels, the quality of the blood flow, and the degree of hemoglobin oxidation.

others have characteristic ones such as the mousy odor of pemphigus vulgaris, the overwhelmingly foul odor of anaerobic streptococcal infection, and the sweetish, mousy odor of gas gangrene. Determine the presence, also, of itching, paresthesia, or loss of sensation.

When lesions are multiple, observe their configuration or arrangement (discrete, annular, linear, grouping). Some configurations are very distinctive, such as linear arrangement along the path of a peripheral nerve in herpes zoster and the annular arrangement of tinea corporis (ringworm).

The distribution of skin lesions over the body may be characteristic or variable for specific disorders. Even when not characteristic, the information can be quite helpful, so look for distribution patterns (bilateral, unilateral; in the creases of joints, folds of tissue; over pressure areas; on exposed surfaces, on protected surfaces).

Emotional trauma can cause a wide variety of skin problems, so a skillful history-taking interview is essential in assessment. The time interval between emotional stress and some dermatologic problems is often predictable: a few minutes in urticaria, 1 to 2 days in dermatitis, and 2 weeks in alopecia areata. Observe especially for conflicts in the patient's interrelationships with others.

A thorough and skillful assessment of the skin and mucous membrane of both dark- and fair-skinned patients provides a broad base of information about a patient's total health status. Combined with associated signs, symptoms and behavior, the information often becomes diagnostic. As a nurse you have the responsibility and usually the opportunity to develop the necessary skills for detecting and describing the skin changes that reflect so clearly your patient's state of health or illness.

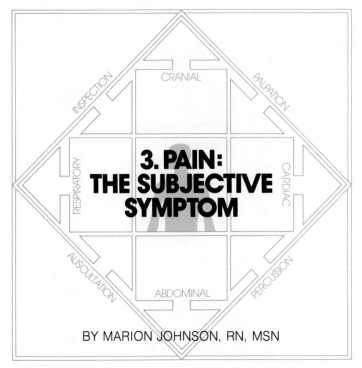

3. PAIN: THE SUBJECTIVE SYMPTOM

BY MARION JOHNSON, RN, MSN

PAIN IS A SYMPTOM — very often the symptom that brings a patient to the physician or hospital. Yet all too often we nurses tend to overlook it as a vital part of assessment. By doing so, we may be bypassing an important clue to the patient's diagnosis.

Of course, individual reactions to pain are highly complex. The patient who grimaces and moans is obviously in pain. But what about the patient who lies motionless in bed, breathing slowly and looking drawn? Or the patient who paces the hall quietly, a look of concentration on his face? Either of them may be in more pain than the first patient.

How, then, can you determine if a patient is in pain? How can you evaluate pain to ensure that the patient receives the kind of care that will, if at all possible, eliminate or ease it? Although there is no one way to assess and evaluate pain for each individual in every situation, you can help if you're aware of some of the pertinent characteristics of pain.

First, pain involves a reaction of the whole personality. Consequently you have to deal not only with the pathophysiology of pain but also with the patient's perception of pain. Thus, though they are interrelated, pain is often de-

Pain's lair

Experts divide chronic pain into six major categories: 1. Muscle and joint pain includes arthritis, bursitis, tendonitis, wryneck, and spinal disk disease and accounts for the greatest number of pain-clinic patients. 2. Causalgia is an intense burning pain that results from trauma to the peripheral nervous system, such as a gunshot wound. 3. Neuralgia arises from a disorder of the peripheral nerves. The most common is trigeminal neuralgia or tic douloureux which affects one side of the face and may be set off by a puff of wind. 4. Vascular pain results from the dilation of blood vessels around the brain. Migraine headaches are the most common example. 5. Terminal cancer pain is produced by tissue destruction and the obstruction of major organs. 6. Phantom limb occurs after amputation and seems to arise from the amputated limb.

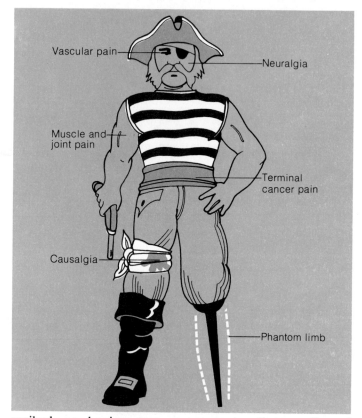

scribed as having two components: "sensory" and "response." You can pinpoint and evaluate the sensory component — or, simply put, the sensation — in terms of where the pain's located, its quality, intensity, and chronology; furthermore, this component has similarities from person to person. The response component, though, can vary markedly among individuals, and is dependent upon psychosocial factors such as personality and cultural background.

Second, there are at least two types of pain, based upon duration — acute and chronic. Acute pain — such as incisional or labor pains — is frequently accompanied by visible signs of discomfort, such as clenched jaws, grimacing, and sweating. Chronic pain, perhaps just as frequently, is not; the patient, for instance, may have lived with his rheumatoid arthritis for so long that he suffers in quiet despair. Unfortunately, despite growing evidence that the signs of acute and chronic pain differ, nurses and doctors typically use acute pain as a model for all kinds and thus can miss a great deal.

As general background in understanding the acute and chronic patient, remember:

• The patient with acute pain generally expects *total* relief since the cause is usually self-limiting or can be corrected. But if this doesn't happen, the letdown can be devastating.

• Acute pain is more frequently accompanied by anxiety than by depression; chronic pain, more often by depression than anxiety.

• Individuals with chronic pain do not become accustomed to it; rather, they may suffer more with the passing of time, as physical and mental depletions occur. Indeed, the smallest amount of additional discomfort may become intolerable.

• The patient with chronic pain may complain of the accompanying fatigue, pleading that he could cope better if he could get a good night's sleep. Unfortunately, most such patients are unable to sleep for prolonged periods.

Determining that pain exists

This might very well strike some of you as too simple even to discuss. "After all," you may be thinking, "who doesn't eventually get to know when someone's in pain? Clues spring up everywhere." Really? Well, research indicates that we know very little about the types of information nurses use to recognize pain. We are learning that nurses don't always rely on the patient's word if he feels pain.

The problem is that, at times, your assessment of a patient's condition may be at variance with what he tells you. Although he may complain that he hurts, you may see none of the usual physical signs of pain — the clenched jaws, the grimacing, the sweating, and so on. On the other hand, he may tell you he's not in pain but you can see from the way he's wincing that he's in anguish. The patient with chronic pain might not even talk about the pain; he might be perceiving the "sensation" differently after so many months or years. For example, a patient might tell you, "Oh, yes, this was painful at first, but I don't think of it as pain any more." But if you don't stop at that, you might learn otherwise. Your patient might be similar to one who stated to me, "No, I'm not having any pain...well, my back is killing me."

So, although you should be alert to the physical indicators

Gate-control theory of pain

A major breakthrough in the study of pain is the gate-control theory (see opposite page) developed by Dr. Ronald Melzack of McGill University and Dr. Patrick Wall of the University of London. The theory, much simplified, goes like this: Sensory receptors throughout the body communicate with the brain via nerve fibers. Large nerve fibers transmit touch impulses which travel to the brain faster than the pain impulses carried by the small nerve fibers. Both sets of nerves converge in the spinal cord where, Wall and Melzack hypothesize, a gate-like mechanism that is usually closed can open to admit sensations. Electrical stimulation, acupuncture, hypnosis, excitement, or pleasure activate the large nerve fibers whose touch impulses beat the pain impulses to the brain and close the gate. Anxiety and apprehension, on the other hand, seem to keep the gate open.

that accompany acute pain, you shouldn't stop there. If a patient tells you he's in pain, assume that he is. Ask him how he feels, but don't rely on the word "pain" when questioning him. Use such words as "hurt" and "discomfort" to bring out different levels of feeling. Observe the patient. Look not only for physical signs but also for *changes* in physiologic signs that may indicate pain. The postoperative patient, for example, may exhibit an elevated blood pressure and pulse even before he is alert enough to report pain. The patient with chronic pain may move around less, stirring only when necessary. In any case, whenever your eyes — or intuition — tell you there may be pain, discuss it with the patient.

Develop an understanding of typical pain patterns. You will find, for example, that pain after abdominal surgery may follow this pattern: Incisional pain may be most severe on the first and second postoperative days and begin to decrease by the third. Deeper visceral and gas pains will become more severe by the third or fourth postop day and may predominate. To help the patient understand what's happening, you must be able to relate the pain to his particular pathology. Not knowing this relationship can make pain a nightmare for the patient.

Assessing the pain

Once you've determined that the patient is in pain, you should evaluate its components: location, intensity, quality, and chronology. Since patients respond to pain subjectively, evaluating it can be extremely difficult. But you may be able to do so with a few questions. Don't use leading questions during the initial evaluation, such as "Is your pain intense? Throbbing? Intermittent?" Instead, have the patient describe his pain in his own words. After he has volunteered as much information as he can, you may *then* need to ask more direct questions.

Assessing the location of the pain is essential for several reasons. For instance, it can prevent incidents in which patients are treated for abdominal pain, because that's what everyone assumes it is, only to find out the pain's in his chest. Have the patient be as specific as possible. Since he may confuse the area of radiation with the point of origin, ask him to trace the area of the pain from its severest point. If the patient can't be precise, have him describe areas that are pain-*free*. You may then learn that the pain is located, say,

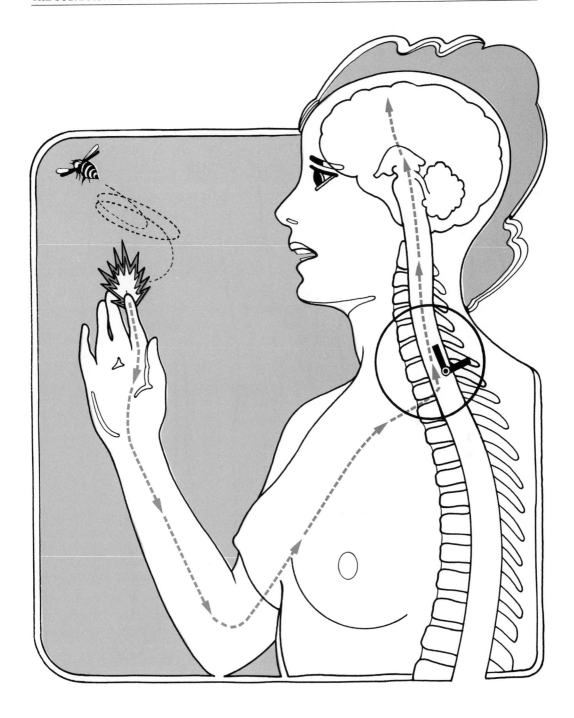

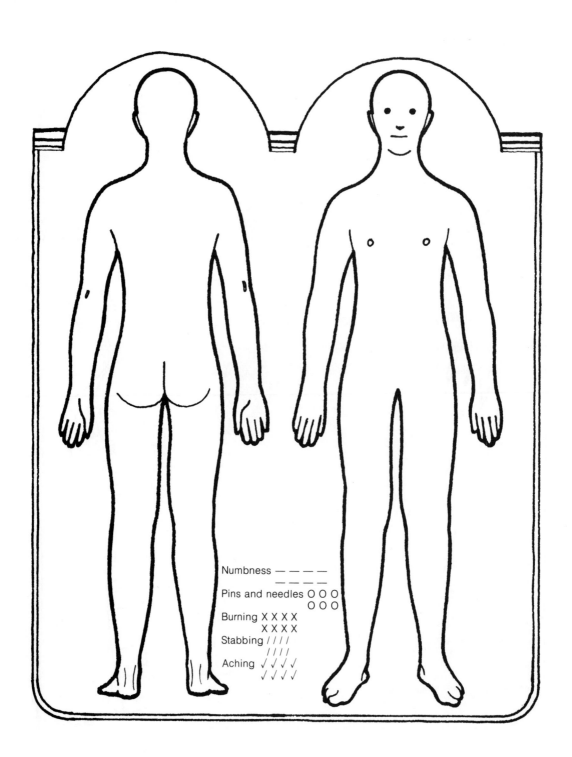

Numbness — — — —
— — — —
Pins and needles O O O
O O O
Burning X X X X
X X X X
Stabbing / / / /
/ / / /
Aching √ √ √ √
√ √ √ √

over the abdominal and pelvic area except for the left upper quadrant. Generally speaking, you can locate superficial or cutaneous pain more precisely than visceral pain (involving body organs) or somatic pain (bone, muscle, and other deep structure).

To assess the intensity of pain, remember the influence of subjectivity. The intensity of the pain doesn't necessarily parallel the importance of the cause: Thus the severe pain of neuralgias can be set off by a slight touch.

You can make your evaluation of intensity more objective by asking the patient to rank the pain; use words such as "mild," "moderate," "severe," and "unbearable." Or you may prefer to use numbers, say, 0 to 10. Try asking the patient how the pain compares with other pains: Is it more severe than a toothache or stomach cramps? In this way you often can pick up clues to the way the patient normally ranks pain. And you can use this comparison scale to determine more easily whether the pain is increasing or decreasing.

To assess the quality, remember that people vary in their verbal abilities. But there is some consistency in the way people describe certain types of pain. Pain caused by an obstructed organ or tube (renal colic, for instance) is often described as "cramping," "twisting"; pain associated with myocardial infarction is often described as "squeezing," "crushing," "binding." Other kinds of pain may not lend themselves to accurate description; visceral pain, for instance, is diffuse and so may be difficult to describe other than as a dull ache or soreness. Here again, allow patients to use their own words. If they're not able to describe the pain, don't simply ask, "Is the pain sharp?" This calls for a yes or no answer that may not be enough. Rather, give them some options such as, "Would you describe the pain as 'cutting,' 'crushing,' or 'burning'?"

The chronology of pain depends on the kind and on how long it lasts. If the following are pertinent and not self-evident, you should probe for:

• The precipitating event. How did the pain start and what caused or precipitated it? Under what circumstances does the patient suffer?

• Any variance between the character of the pain and the time it occurred.

• Duration of the pain and of all alleviating factors. When

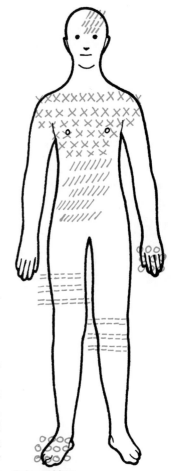

Pains taking
The figure above illustrates how and where one patient perceived his pain. You may wish to copy the chart on the opposite page for your patients to mark with the appropriate symbols.

Numbness — — — —

Pins and needles O O O O

Burning X X X X

Stabbing / / / /

was the onset? Has the patient's pain been steady? Has the nature of it changed? Does distraction help, and if so, of what kind? Does rest (as in the case of angina) bring relief? The clearer a portrait you can give of the character of the pain, the better a diagnosis or treatment the physician will be able to provide.

• Are any other symptoms present? Be alert to any changes in vital signs such as slow pulse or a fall in blood pressure that may accompany visceral pain, or edema and changes in skin color and temperature that you may see with somatic pain. Do what you can to relieve the restless irritability that discomfort may cause. Find out whether the patient wants company or solitude.

• What coping mechanisms help control the pain? Although comfort measures such as reducing noise and distractions will never relieve sharp pain, they may lessen pain or discomfort.

Assessing response component

The patient lies there silently. Perhaps he shows some of the symptoms of pain that occur with stimulation of the sympathetic nervous system, such as dilated pupils, sweating, and increased blood pressure, respiration, and pulse rate. Or he may show evidence of parasympathetic nervous system stimulation, such as a fall in blood pressure, which may occur when pain is severe or the patient near collapse. But though you can surmise that the patient's in pain, you can't truly know if you're correct, or the degree of the pain, or how it's affecting the patient psychosocially unless you communicate with him.

Check his chart. Remember that personality and cultural background influence a patient's response to pain, affecting his pain threshold and how emotional he becomes.

Try to find out:

• How the pain alters his activities — both work and play.

• If the pain has changed or might change his relationship with others.

• What he wants to be able to do. You may control the pain enough to permit him his most important activities.

Also talk with his physician and other nurses.

Remember that you are in a key position to help patients burdened with pain. You can help lift it from them. Or you can lighten it by sharing it with them.

SKILLCHECK 1

1. Emily Jonas, a 55-year-old bookkeeper, has been admitted with a myocardial infarction. The emergency room nurses recorded her vital signs as follows: blood pressure, 110/80; pulse, 72 regular; respiration, 18 regular. After starting Ms. Jonas on 10 mg morphine sulfate I.V. for the chest pain and O$_2$ via cannula, the doctor transferred her to your floor.

Now, three hours after her initial morphine dose, Ms. Jonas still has chest pain. You give her 5 mg morphine I.V. as ordered, which relieves the pain. But suddenly Ms. Jonas becomes nauseated and starts vomiting.

What could have caused the vomiting? What assessments would you make?

2. At midnight, 38-year-old Mark Schwenk is admitted to the hospital after 2 hours of chest discomfort. His vital signs on admission are: blood pressure, 110/70; pulse 55, regular; respiration, 18 regular. Although his signs are normal, the doctor wants to rule out the possibility of myocardial infarction. Since the CCU is full, he sends Mr. Schwenk to your unit.

When Mr. Schwenk arrives, he tells you that his chest pain and shortness of breath have disappeared. What's more, he reassures you, he couldn't have had a "heart attack" because he's in excellent physical condition and once was a champion long-distance runner.

What assessments would you make?

3. Sadie, a 55-year-old housewife, is 2 days post-op after removal and biopsy of a breast cyst. Her incision site appears to be healing well and her vital signs remain stable. But Sadie continues to ask for pain medication every 4 hours.

Her roommate Gwen, a 50-year-old saleswoman, has had her knee replaced because of severe arthritis. Today is her first day post-op. Gwen is very cooperative and denies pain, but she seems very quiet.

How would you assess their behavior?

4. Darlene Brown is a 21-year-old patient who 3 days ago had a bilateral wedge resection for infertility. Since her operation, she has recuperated well. Today, in fact, she spent most of her time out of bed and ambulating. And, she asked for pain medication only once.

When you go to Darlene's room after visiting hours, though, you find her lying on her side, legs pulled up, crying. She says she just wants to go home.

What assessments would you make?

5. While giving Becky Holz a back rub, you notice a small raised area on her mid-back.

How would you handle the situation?

6. Mrs. Rose Serrao, an elderly lady with a history of arteriosclerotic heart disease, has been admitted because she fractured her femur. Her leg is in traction and she is scheduled for surgery early tomorrow morning.

When you check her tonight, she seems restless and unable to sleep, although she doesn't complain of pain.

Before administering her ordered p.r.n. sedation, you check her vital signs and find the following: blood pressure, 156/95; pulse, 110; respiration, 28.

What would you do?

7. Alexander Lincoln, a 49-year-old black man, was brought to the emergency room after collapsing at work. Co-workers said he gasped and grabbed at his chest before collapsing.

Mr. Lincoln has been resuscitated and placed on a cardiac monitor. His vital signs are: blood pressure, 100/60; pulse, 80; respirations, 28. The monitor shows normal sinus rhythm, although periodically you notice some ST segment irregularities.

What skin assessments should you make?

(answers on page 181)

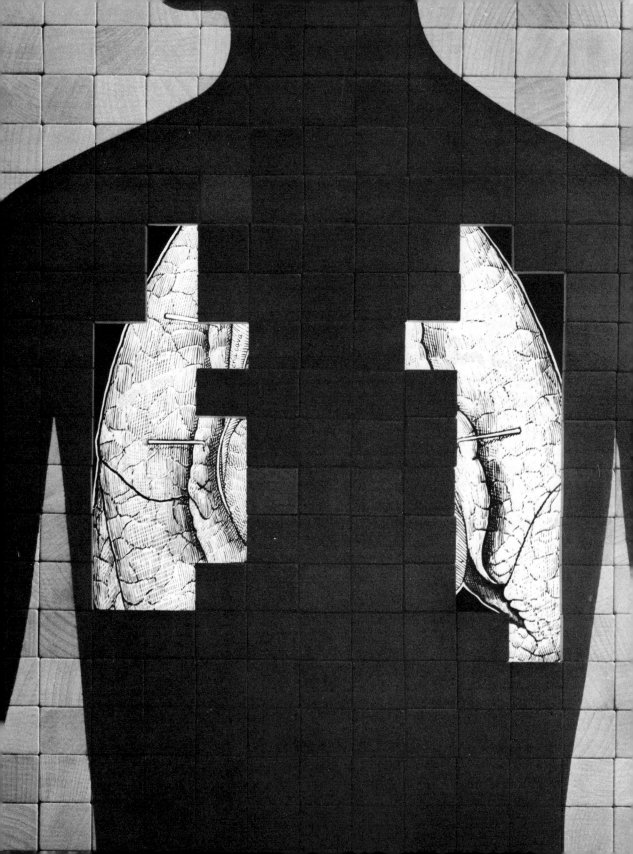

ASSESSING RESPIRATORY FUNCTION

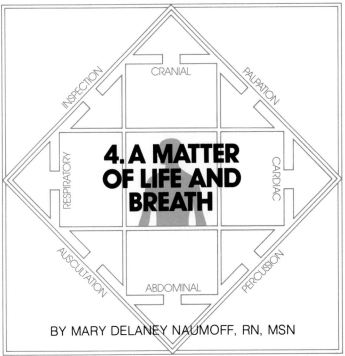

INSPECTION PALPATION
CRANIAL
RESPIRATORY CARDIAC

4. A MATTER OF LIFE AND BREATH

AUSCULTATION PERCUSSION
ABDOMINAL

BY MARY DELANEY NAUMOFF, RN, MSN

SURELY FEW PATIENTS are in a more critical state than the ones whose heart and lungs are compromised by illness. Not only in chest patients but often in others as well, the thorax — the very seat of the blood and breath — holds the key to survival.

Although the secrets of the chest are there to be read, you need skill to do it. And changes can happen fast. When someone is either very ill or on the verge of being so, the chest should be checked often. Since you, rather than the doctor, are with the patient under most circumstances, it's up to you to learn to interpret chest signs — as more and more nurses are doing. In caring for the less seriously ill patient, too, physical examination is an integral part of nursing assessment and evaluation. And these two things in turn are the basis of both planning and performance. In any case, the techniques you develop will stand you and your patients in good stead.

In the next section of this book, you'll learn how to assess the heart. But here let's look at its equally vital counterpart — the lungs. As mentioned in Chapter 1, you'll need four skills to examine the lungs: inspection, palpation, percussion, and auscultation. Used systematically, these techniques can give you

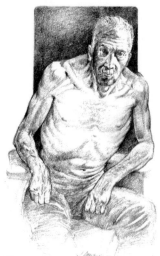

The pink puffer
The posture of the man above is typical of a patient with almost pure emphysema, known as a "pink puffer." Such a patient is generally thin, looks pink, has cardiac enlargement and little sputum production. In contrast, the "blue bloater," a patient with almost pure chronic bronchitis, is often heavyset, appears blue or red-blue around the face, and has ankle edema and distended neck veins.

updated, frequent, and useful clinical information on a patient's respiratory status.

Inspection: Follow a mental checklist
The technique of observing respiration was covered in Chapter 1. When performing this phase of assessment, remember to ask yourself specific questions, such as:
- What are the patient's attitude and general appearance as he lies in bed?
- Is he calm or apprehensive?
- Is he hyperpneic or breathing shallowly?
- What is the color of his skin? Of his mucous membranes?
- Is his thoracic cage moving symmetrically?
- Does he have kyphosis? Scoliosis?
- What muscles does he use to breathe? Diaphragm? Intercostals? Neck and shoulders?
- Is his skin dry or is he diaphoretic?
- How labored are his respirations?

The answers to these questions will often tell you what to look for during the rest of your assessment. For instance, if you see a patient who is cyanotic, has a barrel chest, and is using his auxiliary muscles to breathe, you know immediately that he has poor compliance and decreased perfusion of gases with the alveoli. If you notice localized intercostal retraction, you should check for obstructed bronchi. If you notice localized bulging of intercostal tissue, check for a crushing chest injury. If the patient's chest expands asymmetrically, check for pneumothorax, obstruction of a major bronchus, misplaced endotracheal tube, or unilateral chest pain. If the trachea shifts from the midline to his unaffected side, check for tension pneumothorax; if it shifts to his affected side, check for atelectasis.

Palpation: Need for hands on
Normally you can feel the resonance of voice sounds on the chest with your hands: These vibrations are called fremitus. Start just under the clavicle in front, working down. Like inspection, palpation must be done systematically. You examine both sides of the chest by laying your hands on the skin symmetrically above the scapulae in back, again working down. As you place your hands, have the patient keep saying "99" in a low voice.

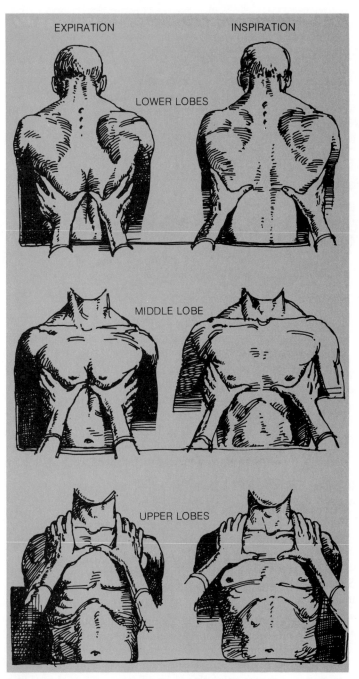

EXPIRATION   INSPIRATION

LOWER LOBES

MIDDLE LOBE

UPPER LOBES

Chest test

To check for symmetrical chest expansion, stand at the foot of the patient's bed and observe him while he's lying supine. Does his chest expand bilaterally with inspiration? Next, lightly place your hands on his chest, first at the bottom of the sternal border and then at the top. Your thumbs should touch the sternal borders when the patient exhales. When he inhales, your thumbs should move equidistant from the sternum. If the patient is prone, use the same procedure with your thumbs touching his spine.

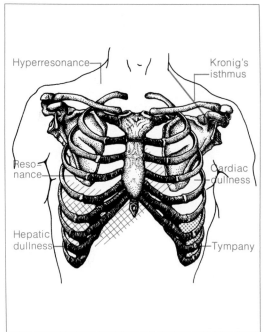

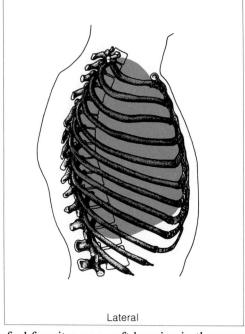

Lateral

Where there is air
These illustrations show the
position of the lungs in relation to
the ribs. You can also see where
different lung sounds originate.

Ordinarily you feel fremitus as a soft buzzing in the upper lobes that decreases to almost nothing in the lower lobes. The significance? Sound is best conducted through solid material, passes less well through water, and least well through air. If the lungs are affected by atelectasis, pneumonia, tumor, or accumulated secretions, you will feel increased fremitus on the affected side. But with emphysema, pneumothorax, or pleural effusion, fremitus will be noticeably decreased or even absent directly over the affected area.

Percussion: Immediate and mediate
Percussion is a difficult skill to learn, but satisfying to know. The two techniques of percussion are: immediate, when you strike your fingertip on the chest wall directly; and mediate, when you lay your middle finger flat on the body and tap it with the first or middle finger of the other hand.

You can best learn percussion by sitting with your arm resting on a flat surface and flexing only your wrist while striking your finger with an opposite finger. Attune your ear to the reverberations that different inanimate surfaces make.

You can hear five sounds in percussion: tympany, hyperresonance, resonance, dullness, and flatness. Only the middle

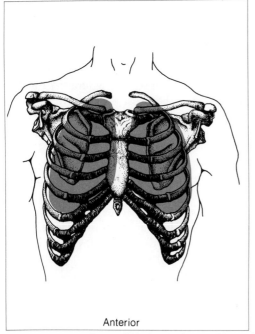

Anterior

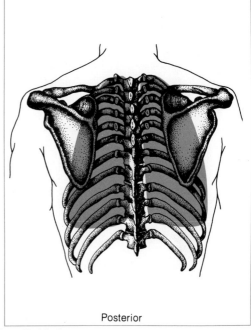

Posterior

three are normally audible in the lungs. You will probably hear tympany over such a gas-filled organ as the stomach, for example, while the reverberation from a large bone — say the scapula — would be flat. In listening to the lungs as you percuss outside them, you would hear hyperresonance over Kronig's isthmus (between the head of the humerus and the base of the neck). Over the same areas where you felt normal fremitus, you should now hear resonance. At the diaphragm and over the heart, percussion will normally sound dull. (See illustration.) But if the lung fields sound dull, the lungs may be consolidated. If they sound too resonant, they may have large air pockets.

Auscultation: Adding a stethoscope

The final step of lung assessment is listening with a stethoscope. As you know, the chest piece of the stethoscope is composed of a bell and diaphragm. The bell, used to discern low-frequency sounds, is a hard cone. It is hollow and smaller in diameter than the diaphragm. The diaphragm, used to detect high-frequency sounds, is a shallow cup that is made of plastic. Only the diaphragm is pressed tightly against the skin. Listen first with the diaphragm in the suprascapular area on the right,

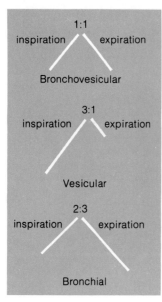

Lengths of breath

and next on the corresponding left side of the chest. Then work your way down to the interscapular region on both sides in order, and finally to the right and left lower lobes.

In the normal lung, the sounds you will hear are bronchovesicular and vesicular, depending on where you listen. You hear bronchovesicular breath sounds where the trachea and the bronchi are closest to the chest wall, above the sternum and between the scapulae. These sounds have two characteristics: The inspiratory and expiratory phases are equal or nearly so; they are a blowing sound of medium to high pitch.

Vesicular breath sounds, those originating in the alveoli, have a soft, breezy quality of medium pitch. Where their inspiratory phase is long, the audible part of expiration is very short; it's only about a third as long as inspiration (see figure).

In early pneumonia these sounds may be lessened, but in late pneumonia, tuberculosis, or if the patient is a heavy smoker, they may be louder than normal. Bronchial breathing is often found in patients with significant atelectasis or consolidation within the lungs. You can imitate this effect by placing the diaphragm of the stethoscope over the trachea. This breath sound is loud and high-pitched; sounds like air blown through a hollow tube; and is longer in the expiratory than in the inspiratory phase, with a short pause between them (see figure).

How to listen: Snap and crackle
Listen first to the upper lobes of the lungs, comparing one side with the other. Ask the patient to take deep breaths with his mouth open. Progress systematically down to the interscapular areas and the lower lobes, always comparing opposite sides. Pay attention to quality, depth, length, and pitch of the inspiratory and expiratory phases.

Sometimes, especially in the acutely ill, you will hear extra or adventitious noises. Most commonly these are rales and rhonchi, bronchial breath sounds, or absent breath sounds.

When you are listening for rales, pay attention to five basic types: musical, crepitant, subcrepitant, bubbling and gurgling. (Rale is French for rattle.) Musical rales may be sibilant, such as the high-pitched wheeze or squeak of an asthmatic attack. Or they may be sonorous or snoring, a low-pitched noise

SITE OF OCCURRENCE

| Bronchi | Bronchioles | Alveoli |

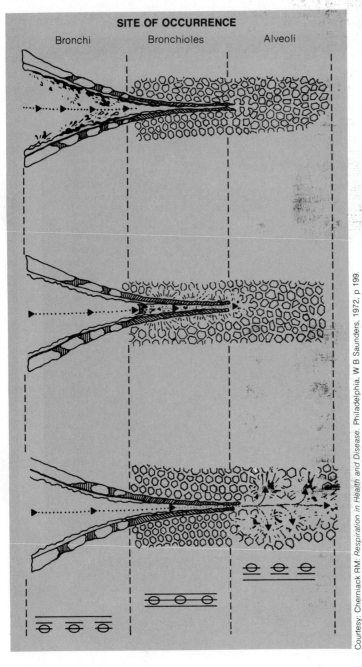

Courtesy: Cherniack RM: *Respiration in Health and Disease.* Philadelphia, W B Saunders, 1972, p 199.

Wheezes, squeaks, crackles, bubbles, and pops

Rales are associated with pulmonary congestion and often indicate imminent heart failure. You can hear rales, usually on inspiration, in the bases of the lungs. The popping sound occurs as air moves through and pops open collapsed airways or parts of the lungs filled with fluid.

SIGNS AND SYMPTOMS IN COMMON LUNG CONDITIONS

CONDITION	INSPECTION	PALPATION	PERCUSSION	AUSCULTATION
Consolidation	Less motion on affected side	Increased fremitus	Dull to flat	Increased intensity of voice and breath sounds; medium to coarse rales on inspiration, friction rub
Pneumothorax	Less motion of respiration on affected side	Decreased fremitus	Hyperresonant	Voice and breath sounds diminished in intensity
Asthma and emphysema	Hyperinflation common; expiration prolonged	Fremitus normal or decreased	Resonant or hyperresonant; motion of diaphragm low and decreased	Voice normal; varied breath sounds possible; wheezing and rhonchi
Pleural effusion	Intercostal spaces on affected side less defined	Decreased fremitus	Flat	Voice and breath sounds diminished in intensity
Atelectasis	On affected side less motion and lowered volume of thorax	Varied fremitus	Dull	Varied voice sounds; breath sounds diminished in intensity; possible bronchial breathing
Congestive failure without effusion	Mostly normal	Normal	Normal	Fine to medium rales louder on right than on left
Bronchitis	Normal	Normal	Normal	Presence of localized rales, rhonchi, and wheezing

caused by air passing through narrowed larger airways. Musical rales can be heard equally well on inspiration and expiration. In fact, they may be so loud as to obliterate the normal breath sounds. Crepitant rales, or fine moist rales, are high-pitched crackles. You can usually hear them best on terminal inspiration, and coughing will not clear them. (To simulate the noise, rub a few hairs together over your ear.) The crepitant rale is a meaningful finding because it most often signifies excess fluid or pus in the alveoli. The usual causes are early pulmonary edema, pneumonia, or tuberculosis.

Initially, crepitant and atelectatic rales may sound alike. The difference is that atelectatic rales, which are frequently heard after patients have been on bedrest or have been splinting their abdomens after surgery, will readily disappear after a few good, deep breaths. Subcrepitant rales, or medium-moist rales, are similar to crepitant rales except that they sound wet and do not crackle or pop. Listen for them on inspiration. They are thought to be caused by fluid in the bronchioles as well as in the alveoli. You are likely to find them in patients with significant accumulated secretions or pulmonary edema. Bubbling rales (coarse and moist) are often referred to as rhonchi. They have a very wet, bubbling sound; they are probably produced by fluid in the major bronchi. You can often hear them in patients with severe bronchitis, bronchiectasis, or resolving pneumonia. Their distinguishing point: They are most commonly heard on expiration. You can also find bubbling rales and subcrepitant rales in some patients after major surgery, or in those who were debilitated before surgery. For these patients, coughing, deep breathing, and positive pressure will be helpful. Auscultation becomes an invaluable tool in evaluating the effectiveness of treatment.

Gurgling rales, often called the death rattle, are wetter than bubbling rales. The patient is usually moribund or too ill to clear secretions from his trachea and right and left bronchi, and these rales are frequently audible without a stethoscope. Gurgling rales are both inspiratory and expiratory.

Other sounds

Bronchial breath sounds, which you will usually hear in the presence of a major atelectasis, unresolved pneumonia, a tumor, or above a pleural effusion, resemble the tracheal breath sounds that you can hear by putting the stethoscope

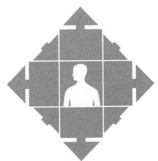

Health history:
What you should know
1. Does the patient have a history of lung disease: pneumonia, tuberculosis, asthma, or frequent colds?
2. Does he smoke? Does his job affect his respiration?
3. Does he suffer from dyspnea, pain, coughing? What are the characteristics of each?
4. When was his last chest X-ray?

diaphragm over the trachea. Absent or diminished breath sounds are the uncharacteristic pulmonary silences that occur either over a massive pleural effusion, in someone with severe chronic obstructive lung disease, or on the side of a pneumothorax.

Planning the patient's care

When you have mastered the systematic examination of a patient's lungs and taken an adequate history from a particular patient, you can collaborate with the physician much more knowledgeably in devising a suitable patient care plan. The information obtained and validated also provides you with the baseline data needed to evaluate your care plan. In addition, using these skills provides the primary data you need to sharpen your clinical judgment and make immediate modifications of the original care plan.

Mastering physical diagnosis of the chest is not as difficult as it may sound. But you will need good eyes, good ears, a stethoscope, your own good common sense, determination, and practice. You will have the satisfaction of having added an important assessment skill.

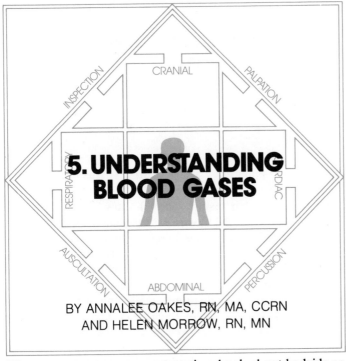

5. UNDERSTANDING BLOOD GASES

BY ANNALEE OAKES, RN, MA, CCRN
AND HELEN MORROW, RN, MN

WHY INCLUDE BLOOD-GAS tests in a book about bedside assessments — particularly about assessments that you can make without monitoring equipment or lab tests? Simply because most hospitals now use blood-gas studies in the care of critically ill patients. Many nurses, however, completed their education before nursing schools began to teach the concepts necessary for understanding blood-gas tests. Without some instruction, you are almost sure to miss the vital information that blood-gas reports can give you — such as whether the patient can meet his oxygen and carbon dioxide needs or requires assistance, and just what assistance to give. This chapter will give you the basics of blood gases.

Here we will discuss mainly the most common blood-gas reports. The following case shows how much these tests can tell you.

Mrs. T., a markedly obese woman in her early forties, was admitted with weakness, somnolence, and ankle swelling that had lasted a year. All had grown progressively worse. Her physical examination showed she was 65 inches tall and weighed 285 pounds. Her breathing was labored and shallow; her nail beds showed cyanosis. X-rays showed enlargement of

LABORATORY RESULTS WERE:		
	Mrs. T.	Normal
PaO$_2$	40 mm Hg	90-95 mm Hg
PaCO$_2$	64 mm Hg	40 mm Hg
HCO$_3^-$	37 mMol/L	24 mMol/L
pH	7.39	7.4
Hemoglobin	20 Gm/100 ml	12-18 Gm/100 ml
RBCs	8.5 million/cu mm	4-6 million/cu mm

the heart and pulmonary arteries. Mrs. T. was breathing ambient air with an oxygen content of 21%.

What did her lab results (above) show? First, Mrs. T.'s arterial oxyen level (PaO$_2$) was less than half the normal figure. She was dangerously oxygen hungry. Her blood carbon dioxide (PaCO$_2$) had increased dramatically. Despite this, her pH acid-base index had remained within a normal range — but only because of an increased bicarbonate blood level (HCO$_3^-$). This bicarbonate retention represented a long-term compensation by the kidneys to correct acidemia. She was actually in chronic, compensated respiratory acidosis, as we shall see later.

Notice that the laboratory report shows elevated levels of both hemoglobin (Hgb) and red blood cells (RBC). The RBC count is twice normal. These values describe the body's remaining mechanism for relieving oxygen lack by increasing the oxygen-carrying capacity of the blood. Such compensation works for awhile — until the blood becomes so viscous that it compromises circulation. Considered with the low oxygen tension (PaO$_2$), the high Hgb and RBC indicate long-standing hypoxemia.

Obviously, Mrs. T. badly needed oxygen therapy, but what percentage of oxygen, at what rate, and for how long? Before answering, let's review the normal respiratory pattern.

In healthy people, the impetus to breathe comes from two stimuli: an elevation of PaCO$_2$ or hydrogen ions (H$^+$), or both, in the brain's medulla. Up to a certain point, an increase in blood CO$_2$ causes faster and deeper ventilation. But some authorities say that levels beyond about 9% or 68 mm Hg create a depressing or narcotic effect on the medulla. This PaCO$_2$ narcosis occurs only in disease, and Mrs. T.'s laboratory values indicated her precarious borderline position. At any moment, the high $PaCO_2$ might begin to lull the principal breathing center, leaving her dependent entirely on the second breathing stimulus, her hypoxic drive. A word of caution is in order at this point. If high concentrations of O_2 were administered and the PaO_2 rose to normal or nearly normal levels, the survival action to breathe would be abolished and Mrs. T. might stop ventilating entirely.

How much oxygen did she require? What $PaCO_2/HCO_3^-$ relationship can be established? Was Mrs. T. acidotic or alkalotic? This is where the whole subject of blood gases comes in. Emphasis here will be on the most used determinations: oxygen and carbon dioxide.

Reviewing atmospheric pressure

Because of gravitational pull, the earth's atmosphere exerts a pressure of 14.7 pounds per square inch at sea level. This pressure is strong enough to support a column of water about 30 feet high or a tube of mercury (Hg) about 30 inches tall — 760 millimeters. To make measurement easier, 760 mm Hg is accepted as the standard. Although barometric pressure falls from 760 mm Hg as altitude increases, all laboratory equipment has been adjusted to compensate and report values accurately.

The earth's atmosphere is made up of a mixture of gases, chiefly 79% nitrogen (N_2) and 21% oxygen (O_2). Each exerts a partial pressure in proportion to the volume present. In reporting blood gases, "P" stands for partial pressure.

Short course in abbreviations

Follow the series of steps for gas exchange in your body by referring to the chart, Respiratory Gas Exchange, on the following page. Values appearing most often in lab reports are boxed.

The abbreviations used in this diagram are standard nomenclature in most textbooks and laboratories. For example, PIO_2 refers to the pressure of oxygen in the inspired air. The "I" means inspired. Likewise, PAO_2 refers to the partial pressure of oxygen in the alveoli. The upper case "A" means alveolar gas; lower case letters indicate gases in the liquid phase, either dissolved in the blood or bound chemically, as

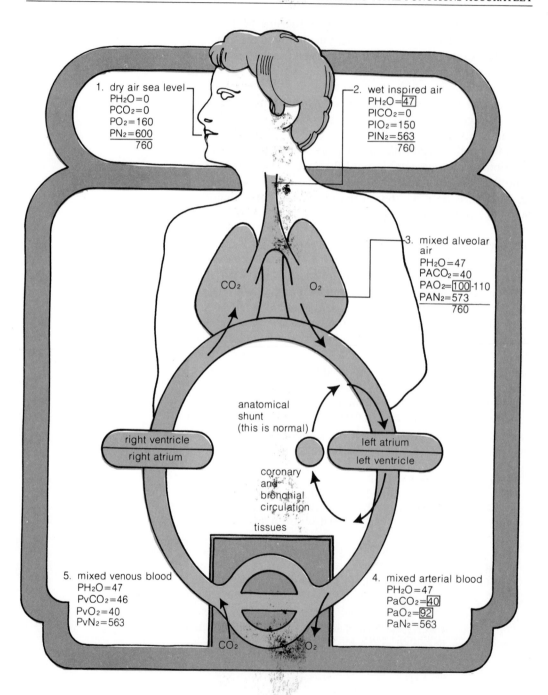

oxygen is bound to hemoglobin. For example, PaO_2 means partial pressure of the oxygen in the arterial blood. The lower case "a" stands for arterial.

Inside story on air

Once air has entered the tracheobronchial tree, water vapor mixes with it immediately. At body temperature and standard pressure, the wet inspired air now contains a partial water vapor pressure (PH_2O) of 47 mm Hg. To maintain an equal air pressure between the lungs and the outside, PH_2O displaces some of the other gases and the PIO_2 becomes 150 mm Hg while the PIN_2 drops to 563 mm Hg. When air finally reaches the alveoli and mixes with the gases there, the oxygen and nitrogen are further reduced by the carbon dioxide returning to the lungs from the right side of the heart. The PAO_2 is then about 110 mm Hg. It is here, across the alveolar membrane, that gas exchange between the lungs and the blood takes place.

In a healthy adult, alveolar and arterial concentrations of carbon dioxide remain at a remarkably constant value — near 40 mm Hg — even during heavy exercise.

The blood from the coronary and bronchial circulations, which comprises approximately 2% of the total circulating volume, returns to the left side of the heart without first going through the lungs for oxygenation. This blood mixes with the oxygenated blood, thereby further reducing the PaO_2 to about 92 mm Hg. These values vary slightly with individuals and laboratory procedures but represent only negligible amounts of oxygen difference, that is, from 90 to 95 mm Hg. Larger variations, however, are indices of clinical conditions.

The other values shown in the chart are those of mixed venous blood and may vary with the metabolic state. For example, a person exercising heavily will have a lower extraction of oxygen PvO_2 value than a less active individual because his skeletal muscles are extracting more oxygen. A person with a fever also will have a low PvO_2 because of his higher metabolic rate.

Hypoventilation confirmed

Comparison of Mrs. T.'s $PaCO_2$ level (64 mm Hg) and her PaO_2 level (40 mm Hg) with the normal levels confirmed hypoventilation from an unknown cause. The elevated $PaCO_2$ was the indicator. Some of the more common reasons for a

Respiratory exchange rate

The illustration on the opposite page shows the pattern of respiratory gas exchange within the human body. Remember that atmospheric pressure is 760 mm Hg; oxygen (O_2) in dry air, 21% or 160 mm Hg partial pressure (PO_2); and nitrogen (N_2) in dry air, 79% or 600 mm Hg partial pressure (PN_2). The boxed numbers in the illustration are especially important.

Knowing nomograms

Some laboratories may not report the bicarbonate (HCO_3^-). If you know the pH and $PaCO_2$, however, you can estimate the HCO_3^-, using the nomogram on the opposite page. Note that the isobars curving upwards from left to right across the page represent various values of $PaCO_2$. The scale at the bottom shows pH values. To find the HCO_3^-, place a straight edge across the chart and locate the intersection of the pH and the $PaCO_2$. This point gives you the HCO_3^- for your patient. In the case of Mrs. T., the intersection of her pH (7.39) and her $PaCO_2$ (64 mm Hg) falls in the shaded area labeled chronic respiratory acidosis across from a HCO_3^- value of 37 milliMol/L.

lower O_2 are congestive heart failure with pulmonary edema, or primary lung disease involving long-term airway obstruction, as in chronic bronchitis or emphysema (see Chapters 4 and 6). Whatever the cause, the effects of the low oxygen tension are obvious.

Oxygen readily combines with hemoglobin even when the partial pressure of oxygen in the blood is low. When the PaO_2 is 92 mm Hg or more, the hemoglobin is 97% saturated. Yet, even at a PaO_2 of 60 mm Hg, hemoglobin is 90% saturated and the patient may still show few signs of oxygen lack. Only at the near-danger level of 50 mm Hg does oxygen dissociate rapidly. Generally too little reserve is left for even simple activities of daily living such as eating and brushing teeth.

Along with retention of CO_2, these patients are sure to demonstrate deprivation of oxygen as did Mrs. T., who deviated from the normal limits because her lungs could not remove the accumulated CO_2 fast enough. She had shifted into respiratory acidosis.

Acid-base balance in brief

To understand Mrs. T.'s chemical shift, let's review acid-base balance. For the normal metabolic reactions to take place, the acid-base balance must be kept within very narrow limits. The nomogram shows the normal blood pH range between 7.38 and 7.44. Acidity is simply an excess of hydrogen ions, alkalinity a deficit. In other words, pH is no more than an expression of hydrogen ion concentration, but since it is shown as a negative logarithm, the numbers in relation to H^+ are the reverse of what you might expect. Where 7.4 is normal, 7 is dangerous, often fatal, acidosis and 7.8, a serious alkalosis. The lungs and kidneys are chief regulators of acid-base chemistry.

If lung function falters, respiratory acidosis occurs from an excess of CO_2. Within a few hours to a week, the kidneys can modify this situation by retaining bicarbonate, a buffer that combines chemically with excess acid or base to modify changes in acid-base balance. Nonetheless, absolute blood levels of both carbon dioxide and bicarbonate may remain elevated even though the pH returns to a 7.38 to 7.44 range.

If the patient hyperventilates, as in hysteria, severe pain, congestive heart failure, or from over-use of mechanical respirators, the $PaCO_2$ will fall to less than 35 mm Hg, and the

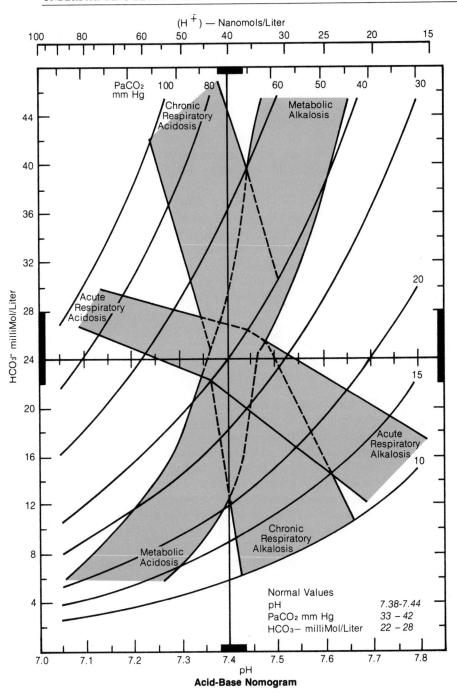

Acid-Base Nomogram

patient is in respiratory alkalosis. Exhaling too much carbon dioxide causes a deficit of H^+ portrayed in the equation by a shift to the left. Respiratory compensation — the patient's re-breathing into a paper bag, for example — can be effective within a few minutes, but is only a stopgap measure and almost never entirely successful. The cause of the hyperventilation should be treated.

Metabolic alkalosis often occurs in the patient who loses hydrochloric acid through severe vomiting or gastric suction. An early sign of this acid-base imbalance is partial respiratory compensation through depressed breathing that consequently increases $PaCO_2$. Later, the bicarbonate level also will be elevated because the kidneys offset the loss of chloride with another anion, HCO_3^-. Medical correction may consist of giving potassium chloride, sodium chloride, or dilute hydrochloric acid, since potassium, sodium and chloride are all depleted. Metabolic acidosis is usually marked by hyperventilation, often by Kussmaul breathing, a paroxysmal hunger for air, and a low $PaCO_2$. In an attempt to reduce high blood concentration of hydrogen ion, the body sacrifices its carbon dioxide. Both diabetic acidosis from excess ketone bodies, lactic acidosis from circulatory compromise, and renal acidosis may cause the above symptoms.

Maintaining a delicate balance
Planning Mrs. T.'s therapy was difficult. To give her no oxygen when the PaO_2 was 40 mm Hg could lower it further, perhaps with irreversible tissue damage. To offer uncontrolled high-flow oxygen might raise the PaO_2 too rapidly and block the hypoxic breathing stimulus.

Of course, in patients so hypoxic that they are confused or even unconscious, you may need to give high concentrations of oxygen — even up to 100% ($PIO_2 = 760$ mm Hg) — until the initial danger is past. When the PaO_2 reaches about 60 mm Hg, adjust the oxygen intake to keep this level steady and raise it thereafter only with monitoring of $PaCO_2$ and PaO_2. Frequent blood-gas measurements are your primary assessment tool in such a case. The absence of cyanosis is not a reliable criterion, and other clinical observations provide only a rough estimate of patient progress. For less critically ill patients, giving 2 to 4 liters of oxygen per minute is usually safe, and many patients can be maintained this way.

METABOLIC/RESPIRATORY — ACIDOSIS/ALKALOSIS
A COMPARATIVE ANALYSIS

	DEFINITION:	PROBABLE CAUSE:	RECOGNITION:	LABORATORY TESTS:
METABOLIC ACIDOSIS	Excess of acid (H^+) and deficit of base (HCO_3^-)	Ketoacidosis: incomplete metabolism of fats (diabetes); renal acidosis; retention of inorganic, phosphoric and sulfuric acids (renal failure); lactic acidosis: incomplete metabolism of CHO; HCO_3^- deficit (diarrhea)	Headache, nausea, vomiting, diarrhea, sensorium changes, tremoring, convulsions	$ph < 7.35$ serum $CO_2 < 22$ mEq/L $pCO_2 < 40$ mm Hg if compensating PO_2 usually normal serum potassium elevated
RESPIRATORY ACIDOSIS	Excess of carbonic acid (H_2CO_3) and elevated $PaCO_2$	Hypoventilation: retention of CO_2, i.e., COPD; muscular weakness	Decreased ventilation, sensorium changes, somnolence, semicomatose-comatose, tachycardia, arrhythmia	$pH < 7.35$ serum $CO_2 > 27$ mEq/L if compensating $PCO_2 > 40$ mm Hg PO_2 usually normal or low; serum potassium elevated
METABOLIC ALKALOSIS	Deficit of H^+ and excess of base (HCO_3^-)	Gastric losses via vomiting, stomach tube, lavage, potent diuretics	Nausea, vomiting, diarrhea, sensorium changes, tremoring, convulsions	$pH > 7.45$ serum $CO_2 > 27$ mEq/L $PCO_2 > 40$ mm Hg if compensating PO_2 usually normal; serum potassium decreased; serum chloride decreased
RESPIRATORY ALKALOSIS	Deficit of carbonic acid (H_2CO_3)	Hyperventilation from neurogenic cause, brain trauma, ventilators	Tachypnea, sensorium changes, numbness, tingling of hands and face	$pH > 7.45$ serum $CO_2 < 22$ mEq/L if compensating $PCO_2 < 40$ mm Hg pO_2 usually normal; serum potassium decreased; urine alkaline

Courtesy: Stroot, Lee, and Schaper. Fluids and Electrolytes: A Practical Approach. Philadelphia, F.A. Davis, 1974. P. 103-105.

Buffering with bicarbonate

Because they cannot readily deal with hydrogen ions per se, the lungs do the next best thing: Each regulates whatever hydrogen ions most easily combine with or dissociate from the body's chemical buffer systems. For example:
$$CO_2 + H_2O \rightleftharpoons H_2CO_3 \rightleftharpoons H^+ + HCO_3^-$$
This equation means that volatile carbon dioxide (regulated by the lungs) plus water yields carbonic acid, hydrogen ion, and bicarbonate ion, which is nonvolatile and regulated by the kidneys. The arrows show that the reaction can proceed in either direction. Bicarbonate is the easiest buffer to measure and it accurately reflects changes in other buffer systems as well.

In the case of Mrs. T., emergency oxygen therapy of 8 to 10 L/min (for 15 to 20 minutes) was replaced with 3 to 4 L/min when she was transferred to a general hospital unit. Complications of pneumonia and overweight slowed the eventual return to normal of her PaO_2. Antibiotics successfully treated the respiratory infection, and long-term therapy included an 800-calorie-a-day diet. By the end of the year, she was 60 pounds lighter, much better, and still dieting.

Monitoring blood gases is not a one-time thing, to be done at the beginning of the patient's hospital stay and then forgotten. After all, blood gases can and do change quickly, particularly in patients with serious conditions. Some doctors, in fact, recommend that nurses check blood gases as often as every 15 minutes after an arrest or other crisis to pick up the very earliest signs of change. Blood gases can guide you when you administer oxygen. Furthermore, when correlated with skilled administration of electrolytes, they can help you prevent wide, dangerous fluctuations in acid-base balance.

In short, using blood-gas findings along with your own assessments can lead to better nursing judgments in the care of your patients.

SKILLCHECK 2

1. Mrs. Rasmussen rushes into the emergency room carrying her unconscious 3-year-old child in her arms. She says her child was playing quietly when he started breathing noisily, turned blue, and lost consciousness.

What immediate assessments would you make?

2. Felix Wonder, a thin 72-year-old, has been admitted for herniorraphy. He has smoked 2 packs of cigarettes a day for 50 years. He received a sleeping pill as ordered at 10 p.m. and slept well until 2 a.m. Now, though, he is awake and becoming progressively noisier and less cooperative. He complains of difficulty breathing and tries to get out of bed. When you check his vital signs, you find that his respiration is 32, his pulse is 110 and irregular, and his blood pressure is 180/100.

What findings can you expect in COPD?

3. Marty Green, who had an abdominal hysterectomy three days ago, now complains of chest pain and dyspnea. When she coughs, she expectorates mucus tinged with blood. Her blood pressure is 120/80, her pulse is 125, her temperature is 101°, and her respiration is 28.

How would you continue this assessment?

4. Peter James, age 28, is admitted to the hospital following an automobile accident in which he was the driver. His extensive facial lacerations have been sutured, and he is now being admitted to your unit. While taking his vital signs you notice diminished movement of the anterior chest wall during inhalation, especially on the right. When questioned he admits to right anterior chest pain that he didn't complain of earlier because he was dazed.

Using the four methods of assessment, how would you evaluate Peter's condition?

5. Joseph Cash, a 65-year-old man, collapsed in a busy shopping mall where a passerby gave him immediate cardiopulmonary resuscitation. Paramedics bringing him to the hospital obtained an arterial blood sample for acid-base determination. The specimen was packed in ice and processed immediately. The results were: pH 7.2; $PaCO_2$, 70; PaO_2, 55; HCO_3^-, 26 mMol/L.

Using the acid-base nomogram, identify Mr. Cash's acid-base status. Describe how you arrive at your diagnosis. What clues in the patient's history support your decision?

6. Two days after Mr. Cash was transferred to the ICU and placed on a volumetric respirator, you note a deteriorating change in his condition. Any tactile stimuli causes Mr. Cash to override the eight breaths/minute respirator setting with tachypneic episodes exceeding 40 per minute. His ventilations are shallow, irregular, and choppy with unilateral chest excursions.

When you auscultate, you hear rales and rhonchi in the right posterior lung base but no breath sounds anywhere over the left chest. You discover his arterial blood gases are pH 7.57; $PaCO_2$, 25; and PaO_2, 50. His chest X-ray findings show infiltration of the left lower lobe and extension of the tip of the endotracheal tube into the right mainstem bronchus.

Using the acid-base nomogram, identify the missing HCO_3^- data and Mr. Cash's current acid-base status.

7. Ian Parker, a 59-year-old man with a smoking history of three packs a day for 40 years, has been admitted to the hospital for gastric resection. After surgery, he has a nasogastric tube and an I.V. On his third morning post-op, he seems lethargic. When he coughs, he brings up ½ a teaspoon of thick yellow sputum.

What assessments would you make?

(answers on page 182)

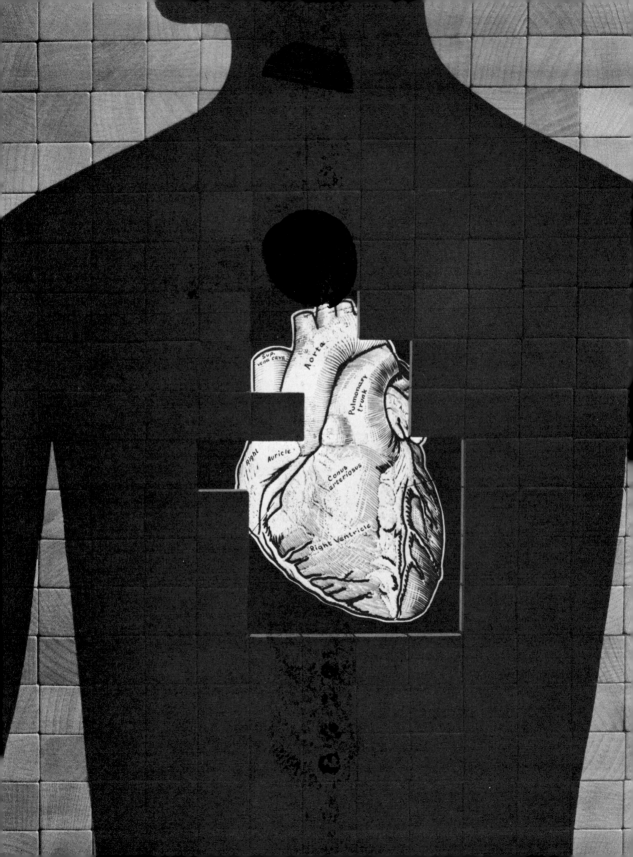

ASSESSING CARDIAC FUNCTION

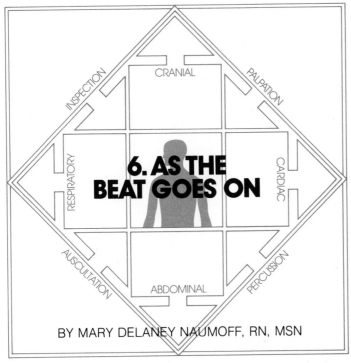

INSPECTION
PALPATION
CRANIAL
RESPIRATORY
CARDIAC
AUSCULTATION
PERCUSSION
ABDOMINAL

6. AS THE BEAT GOES ON

BY MARY DELANEY NAUMOFF, RN, MSN

TRUE, TO DETECT AND monitor the most subtle abnormalities in cardiac function, you have to rely on electrocardiography (see the *Nursing Skillbook* READING EKGs CORRECTLY). But to detect most other cardiac abnormalities, you can rely simply on your basic assessment techniques: Inspection, palpation, percussion, and auscultation, all performed in a cephalocaudal approach. When examining the heart externally, don't forget to keep taking the pulse and blood pressure as well. Both are themselves an excellent index to the state of the circulation.

Inspection: The first clues to serious disorders
Begin with the head and neck. Notice the color of the patient's skin and mucous membranes, his ease or difficulty in breathing, his general demeanor. Pay particular attention to the venous pulsations in the neck, as described in Chapter 1. Raise the head of the bed to a 35° or 45° angle to see if neck veins are distended. Is there obvious arterial-venous pulsation?

When you look at the chest, do you see a precordial heave? That is, does a major portion of the left anterior chest move with the beating of the heart?

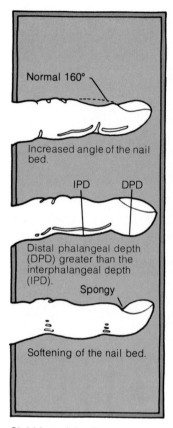

Normal 160°

Increased angle of the nail bed.

IPD   DPD

Distal phalangeal depth (DPD) greater than the interphalangeal depth (IPD).

Spongy

Softening of the nail bed.

Clubbing of the fingers

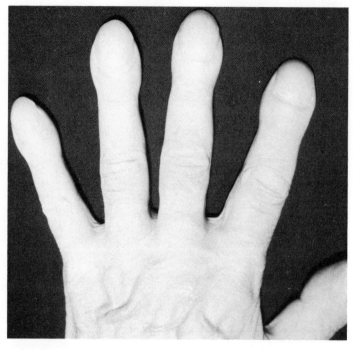

Is there any sign of peripheral edema? If the patient is on bedrest, this may be found only in the sacral area.

All or any one of these cues may be the first intimation of congestive heart failure. They begin to form a picture, although dyspnea at rest may not as yet be evident. Of course, if there are none of these signs, there *could* still be early failure.

Assess the nutritional quality of the hair, skin, and extremities. Nutritional deficiencies coming from insufficient circulation can produce dry, brittle hair, dry skin with keratotic patches, and thickened nails (especially on the toes).

The nails may even be clubbed. The exact cause isn't known. But they are often found in patients with cancer of the lung, chronic lung disease, and congenital cardiovascular disease. And how is clubbing distinguished from familiar roundness of the nails? There are three specific criteria. As shown in the above illustrations, it can be clubbing if:

- the angle between nailbed and finger is greater than 160°;
- the distal phalangeal depth is greater than the depth at the interphalangeal joint;
- the nail bed is unusually soft or spongy.

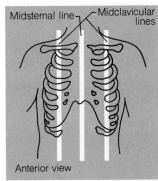

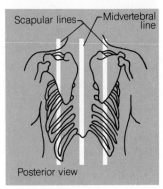

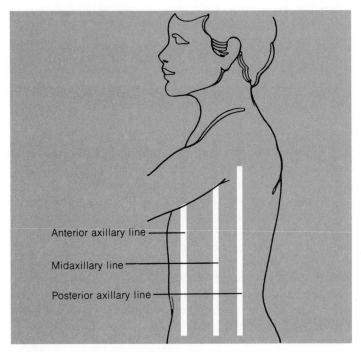

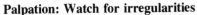

Chest landmarks

Palpation: Watch for irregularities

Now assess the peripheral pulses as described in Chapter 1. Note their rate, quality, and equality. Feel and study the extremities for any noticeable change of color or temperature. And look to see whether hair is obviously missing from the skin. If you suddenly encounter coolness, pallor, or even cyanosis in an extremity along with hairless skin, it may mean an insufficient blood supply from peripheral vascular disease.

Next, concentrate on the anterior of the chest over the precordium. Find the point of maximal impulse (PMI) by palpation. The PMI is usually found in the fifth intercostal space within the midclavicular line (see accompanying figure). Normally you will feel it as a single impulse. Whenever you feel either a double or a paradoxical impulse, you should suspect myocardial pathology that could lead to congestive failure. Note also any irregularity in rate or quality and correlate it with other observations about that patient.

Percussion: How big-hearted

Percussion will help you determine heart size. In the normal

Easy listening

If you are just beginning to learn auscultation or want to refresh your skill, here's a list of heart sound recordings:

Cardiac auscultation
Service of
Merck Sharp & Dohme
West Point, Pa. 19486

Heart sounds
ACCEL Tape
American College of Cardiology
9650 Rockville Pike
Bethesda, Md. 20014

Index of heart sounds and murmurs
National Medical Audiovisual Center
Video Duplication Service
1600 Clifton Road, N.E.
Atlanta, Ga. 30333

Recording of stethoscopic heart sounds
Service of Roerig
Division of Pfizer, Inc.
235 E. 42nd St.
New York, N.Y.10017

Stethoscopic heart record, heart recordings
Columbia 91B02058
(Collector Series)
Columbia Special Products
51 West 52nd St.
New York, N.Y. 10019

adult, the left cardiac border is near the PMI, usually at or within the midclavicular line (MCL).

Percussion techniques used in examining the heart are the same as those for examining the lungs. With the patient lying down, begin to percuss his chest at the anterior axillary line (AAL). Start at the fifth intercostal space (ICS) and move to the fourth if necessary, percussing toward the sternum until you hear dullness. When you hear a change in the note, you have found the left border of cardiac dullness (LBCD). In the average adult male this is usually 10-12 cm from the midsternal line, and always within the midclavicular line. If the LBCD is greater than 12 cm from midsternum and outside the MCL, the heart may be enlarged. Only in a highly trained athlete can this be considered a normal finding.

If you have noticed anything abnormal so far, set out to confirm it through auscultation.

Auscultation: One sound at a time

The key to successful auscultation of the heart is to listen to one sound at a time. You should use both the bell and the diaphragm for examining the heart. (But don't press the bell so hard that it flattens out the skin and in effect becomes a diaphragm.)

Each heart valve sound is reflected to a specific area of the chest wall. In the accompanying figure, you will see that the aortic valve is best heard in the patient's second right ICS and just to *your* left of the sternum. The pulmonic valve is best heard in the patient's second left ICS, just to *your* right of the sternum. The tricuspid valve's reflection of sound will be loudest in the patient's fifth right ICS near the sternum or even in the midline below it, and the mitral valve's reflection of sound will be loudest in the patient's fifth left ICS near the midclavicular line. This last approximates the PMI.

You will need to learn how to distinguish heart sounds through the stethoscope, but with practice you can obtain much valuable information.

Heart sounds: Lubs and rubs

Everyone is familiar with the faithful *lub-dup* of the heart valves. Through the stethoscope you can hear them very clearly; in most charts they are described as S_1 and S_2.

S_1, the first heart sound, is the closing of both atrioventricular valves, the mitral and the tricuspid, just before ventricular systole. (These valves prevent regurgitation of blood into the atria.) The peripheral pulse will occur between the first and second heart sounds. The S_1 sound is the *lub* of *lub-dup*.

The second sound, S_2, is the closing of both semilunar valves, the aortic and the pulmonic, just before diastole — the process of relaxation and refill. These valves serve to prevent backflow into the ventricles. S_2 is the *dup* of *lub-dup*.

The sounds of S_1 and S_2 will differ in loudness as you listen at each valve location. To listen and assess systematically, begin at the apex of the heart by listening to the mitral and tricuspid valves for S_1. Then move to the base over the aortic and pulmonic valves for S_2. Actually, where you start does not make as much difference as doing it the same way every time. This will give your ear the experience it needs.

You may hear unusual or abnormal sounds: rubs, clicks, snaps, splits, hums, crunches, murmurs. When you are making the first assessment of patients, it may be a good idea to refer them all to a doctor or the charge nurse until you are able to distinguish one sound from another and know their significance.

Before you refer murmurs, try to evaluate them and record their location, timing, quality, intensity, and pitch. Murmurs are graded I through VI. The faintest one to be heard is a Grade I murmur. You can hear a Grade VI without a stethoscope.

As you listen with the stethoscope, note carefully:

- The rate and rhythm of the heart.
- The quality of the first heart sound. Is it normal, accentuated, or diminished for that location?
- The quality of the second heart sound. Is it normal, accentuated, or diminished?
- Then compare the second sound at the aortic valve (A_2) with the second sound at the pulmonic valve (P_2). In normal young adults, A_2 is louder than P_2, but in older individuals they are equal. An accentuated second sound at the pulmonary valve — that is, one louder than the A_2 sound — may mean pulmonary hypertension.
- Having compared the S_1 and S_2 sounds, now listen for extra sounds. A third heart sound — S_3 — comes early in diastole if it is present. It is a ventricular flow sound that usually occurs in a dilated ventricle and is caused by the rapid return of blood from the vena cava. You can hear it best at the

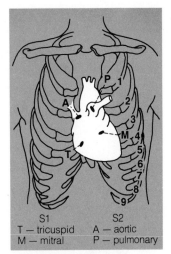

S1
T — tricuspid
M — mitral

S2
A — aortic
P — pulmonary

The doors of the heart
As the figure above shows, the closing of both the atrioventricular (tricuspid and mitral) valves right before ventricular systole produces the sound S_1. The closing of the semilunar (aortic and pulmonary) valves before diastole produces the sound S_2.

apex through the bell with the patient lying on his left side. In a slower heart, S_3 sounds like the "y" in Kentucky. In tachycardia, S_1, S_2, and S_3 sound like a galloping horse; thus the term, "gallop rhythm." S_3 can be perfectly normal in a child or adolescent, or even in a young adult with an extremely thin chest wall. In any other adult it probably means left ventricular failure.

A fourth heart sound, called S_4, may also be heard: Some say it sounds like the "Tenn" in Tennessee. It is an atrial flow sound occurring late in diastole (atrial kick). It is best heard under the same conditions as S_3.

S_4 is an atrial gallop, S_3 a ventricular one. As you are listening, S_3 occurs (if it does) just after S_2; S_4 occurs just before S_1. A summation gallop, combining S_3 and S_4, is a loud single sound that occurs in mid-diastole. An S_3 and a summation gallop should be brought to a physician's attention at once.

Putting your skills to work

What your chest patients need the most are frequent assessment and nursing measures to correspond to their changing condition. If you can examine a chest competently, you can give them this kind of care. You are able to alert the physician to changes in the chest, so that he will have the data he needs to judge and perhaps adjust the patient's regimen.

But don't be discouraged if you don't learn the whole approach at once. It takes a lot of patients — and patience. Here is a case that puts together the patient's history and emphasizes the nurse's skills in recognizing the interdependence of the body's systems.

Mrs. N., 71, was an emergency admission to the hospital, in acute distress from both pulmonary edema and anasarca (massive generalized edema). A widow for the past 13 years, she lived alone in her own home. Just before her admission in January, she had prepared Christmas dinner for her children and their families, numbering 42 in all. I met her 2 days after admission.

For the past year, Mrs. N. had experienced dyspnea after walking as little as one-half block. During the past 6 months her condition had worsened; she had paroxysmal nocturnal dyspnea (PND).

She had suffered a CVA in 1967 that left residual numbness

HOW VARIOUS CAUSES OF CHEST PAIN DIFFER

	MYOCARDIAL INFARCTION	PERICARDITIS	ANGINA	PLEURO-PULMONARY	ESOPHAGEAL-GASTRIC	MUSCULAR-SKELETAL
ONSET	Sudden	Sudden	Build up of intensity (crescendo), or sudden	Gradual or sudden	Gradual or sudden	Gradual or sudden
LOCATION	Substernal; anterior chest, and midline	Substernal, to left of midline or precordial only	Substernal, not sharply localized; anterior chest	Over lung fields to side and back	Substernal, anterior chest; midline	To side of midline
RADIATION	Down one or both arms, to jaw, neck or back	To back or left supraclavicular area	To back, neck, arms, jaw and occasionally upper abdomen, or fingers	Anterior chest, shoulder, neck	To upper abdomen, back, or shoulder	
DURATION	At least 30 min.; usually 1-2 hrs.; residual soreness 1-3 days	Continuous. May last for days. Residual soreness	Usually less than 15 min. and not more than 30 min. (average: 3 min.)	Continuous for hours	Continuous for short or longer intervals, or intermittent	Continuous or intermittent
QUALITY-INTENSITY	Severe, "stabbing," "choking," "squeezing," "vise-like"; intense pressure, deep sensation	Sharp, "stabbing," "knife-like"; moderate to severe or only an "ache"; deep or superficial	Mild to moderate, heavy pressure, "squeezing," "vise-like"; vague, uniform pattern of attacks, deep sensation, tightness	Sharp "ache," not severe; "knife-like," "shooting"; deep; crushing	Squeezing, "heart burn"	Soreness
SIGNS AND SYMPTOMS	Apprehension, nausea, dyspnea, diaphoresis, dizziness, weakness, pulmonary congestion, increased pulse, decreased BP, gallop heart sound, fatigue	Precordial friction rub, muscle movement and inspiration causes increased pain. Pain decreases on sitting or leaning forward, increases when on left side, laughing or coughing	Dyspnea, diaphoresis, nausea, desire to void. Associated with belching, apprehension, or uneasiness	Dyspnea; tachycardia; apprehension; increasing pain with coughing, on inspiration and on movement; pain decreased on sitting. Pleural rub; fever	Dysphagia, belching, diaphoresis, reflux esophagitis, pain decreases on sitting or standing; vomiting	Pain increases with movement
PRECIPITATING FACTORS	Not necessarily anything. May occur at rest or with increased physical or emotional exertion	Not induced with effort	Exertion; stress; eating; cold or hot, humid weather; recumbency; micturition or defecation	Pneumonia or other respiratory infection	Food intake, recumbency, alcohol ingestion, highly seasoned foods, history of GI problems	History of previous neck and arm pain

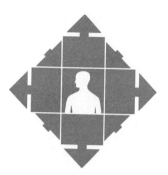

Health history:
What you should know
1. Has the patient a history of heart murmurs, rheumatic fever, or venereal disease? Are any previous injuries, illnesses, surgeries, or treatments relevant to his present condition?
2. Does he suffer from pain, dyspnea, palpitations, fainting, fatigue, or cyanosis? Has he allergies?
3. Do his habits affect his health?
4. Is his family's health history relevant to his present condition?

in the fingers of the left hand but no loss of function. Mrs. N. denied syncope, vertigo, history of rheumatic fever, or previous knowledge of heart disease. She had had a long history of hypertension, which was designated a Class III. During the past 3 months, she had experienced severe anorexia, with a nondeliberate weight loss of 45 pounds.

Physical assessment
Inspection: Mrs. N. was acutely ill, poorly nourished, diaphoretic, and ashen at rest although receiving 4 liters of O_2/min, via cannula.

Her skin was pendulous and cool, with patchy keratoses; bilateral xanthelasmas at the inner canthi of the eyes (indicative of hypercholesterolemia) and 3+ peripheral pitting edema. Neck veins were distended at the angle of the jaw.

Palpation: Liver was 12 cm below right costal margin (see Chapter 9). Fremitus was markedly increased bilaterally in the lower lobes of the lungs. There was marked precordial heave with PMI at the AAL.

Percussion: Dullness over the upper lobes and flatness over the lower lobes. The LBCD began at the AAL and extended 18 cm to the midsternal line (MSL).

Auscultation: Breath sounds: There were crepitant and subcrepitant rales throughout the superior lobes and the middle lobe. Breath sounds were markedly diminished in the superior segments of the lower lobes and absent at the bases of the lungs.

Heart sounds: Heart rate 120/min, regular, but of uneven quality and gallop rhythm. There was marked accentuation of A_2 and it was greater than P_2. An S_3 was clearly audible over the PMI and a III/VI systolic and diastolic murmur was heard over the aortic valve and along the left sternal border (LSB). BP was 120/100.

Inferred medical diagnosis: Acute congestive heart failure. Nursing diagnosis:
• Poor nutritional state from generalized circulatory insufficiency;
• Inability to diffuse gases properly because of pulmonary edema;
• Acute dyspnea from decreased compliance of lung parenchyma because of pulmonary edema;
• Inability to utilize ingested calories adequately because of

decreased available oxygen and moderate hepatic insufficiency.

Based on the data obtained from this first assessment, the following nursing care plan was made:

1. Recommended that her furosemide (Lasix), a diuretic, be increased from 80 mg to 120 mg;

2. Changed from three to five small meals per day. She was already on a 2 Gm sodium diet;

3. Maintained continuous oxygen at 4 liters per nasal cannula;

4. Discussed with the nursing staff how the patient's energy could be conserved and why she should not be coughed to increase her ventilatory capacity.

Two days later Mrs. N. was feeling much better. She had lost 20 pounds of fluid since her first assessment. For the first time in months she was able to sleep all night in bed instead of sitting up in a chair.

Her physical assessment revealed:

Lungs: Crepitant rales were present only in the lower lobes. Breath sounds were audible in the left base although still absent in the right. Respirations were 16/min with no obvious dyspnea.

Heart: No change from the previous findings but the rate had decreased to 90/min and it was in normal sinus rhythm. The S₃ was still faintly present. The liver remained 12 cm below the right costal margin.

Mrs. N. stayed in the hospital another 2 weeks. As she continued to show improvement, her nursing orders were modified accordingly.

On February 5, the day of discharge, she had another complete physical assessment in order to have baseline data for a later home visit.

Lungs: Completely clear to auscultation and percussion with a respiratory rate of 14/min. There was no evidence of dyspnea from walking in the hall. There had been no PND for the past 2 weeks.

Heart: The precordial heave had diminished; heart rate was 70/min and in NSR with a faint S₃ at the apex. BP 140/90.

Liver: Had decreased to 5 cm below right costal margin.

Extremities: No peripheral edema, and 1+ peripheral pulses could be palpated.

The nursing prescriptions upon discharge were:

1. Diet: 1200 calories, 200 mg cholesterol, 2 Gm salt.

2. She was to stay with her daughter for 2 or 3 weeks until her activity tolerance had increased to where she could care for herself at home.

3. She was to rest in bed for 1 hour each morning and afternoon and to sleep 8-10 hours per night. She was not to climb stairs.

4. The purpose and side effects of furosemide, digoxin (Lanoxin), and methyldopa (Aldomet) were explained to Mrs. N. and her daughter.

At home 5 days later, Mrs. N.'s lungs were still clear, and her blood pressure and heart rate remained the same. All of the physical findings were the same as on the day of discharge with one exception: The faint S_3 had now become a loud summation gallop. This very loud flow sound occurs when the S_4 and S_3 are both present; the quadruple rhythm becomes one mid-diastolic sound, usually in the presence of an increased heart rate.

Her attending physician admitted her to the hospital that same day. Her second admission was uncomplicated and she progressed well. Surprisingly, she did not develop acute congestive heart failure and the summation gallop disappeared in 2 days, with the S_3 disappearing in 5 days. Mrs. N. was discharged 10 days after admission. She was visited at home 3 days after discharge and was doing well. Her hypertension was controlled, breath sounds were clear, and there was no evidence of ventricular gallop.

This case history shows how a nurse clinician can plan, evaluate, and modify patient care. With your own increased skill and knowledge, your clinical judgment is sharpened. And you can communicate better with the physician. When you share a common scientific language, the patient's care can be expedited, and the patient benefits.

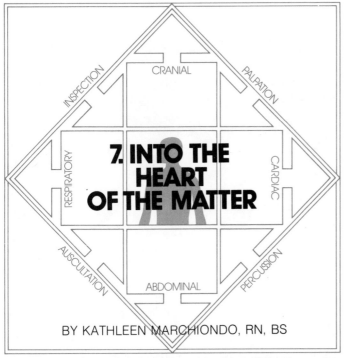

7. INTO THE HEART OF THE MATTER

BY KATHLEEN MARCHIONDO, RN, BS

IN MOST CASES, your routine assessment of the heart (see Chapters 1 and 6) will tell you a patient's cardiac function. But not always. In clinical conditions involving instability in blood volume, cardiac efficiency, or vascular tone, you have to go deeper — deep, in fact, into the heart itself. And one way to do that is with a catheter into the right atrium to measure central venous pressure (CVP).

No matter where you work, chances are you'll have to use this delicate diagnostic tool sometime. Doctors commonly order CVP readings to plan and evaluate care for patients with serious illnesses (such as shock, heart failure, massive myocardial infarction, hemorrhage, coronary occlusion with shock, and undetermined oliguria and anuria) and for patients undergoing intricate procedures (such as cardiac and other major surgery, renal dialysis, coronary arteriography, and cardiac catheterization).

Unlike arterial blood pressure, which is measured in millimeters of mercury, the much lower CVP is measured in centimeters of water. The scientific principle is simple. A column of water will flow from a higher pressure area to one that is lower — until the forces equalize. The CVP monitor is

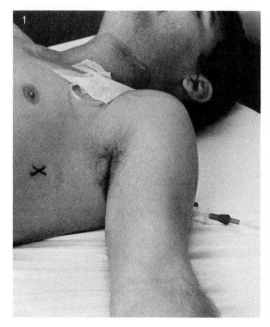

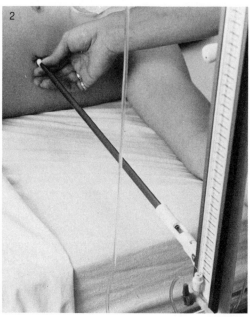

Meaningful monitoring
To take CVP readings correctly, you should adopt a strict procedure, then follow it each time. The photos shown here, and described in the accompanying text, show steps most authorities recommend to eliminate error and complications.

basically a column of water with a capacity of about 30 cm. When its stopcock is opened so that flow is directed into the patient, the column of water recedes downward until it meets the venous pressure.

After the doctor has inserted the CVP catheter (usually in the superior or inferior vena cava), your job is to measure and level the manometer, take periodic readings, and accurately interpret data — always guarding against complications.

How do you get a reading?

Before taking a reading, make sure the bed is level. If the doctor has ordered the patient's head elevated for some reason, such as chest surgery, just make sure it is elevated at the same height for each CVP reading. And if the patient has just undergone some painful procedure, wait until he relaxes.

Check the system. The 3-way stopcock should be turned so that the fluid drips into the vein. (When the pressure is not being taken, the slowly dripping solution keeps the needle open.) Also make sure the manometer is correctly placed in respect to the patient's body. To do this, place the "O" mark of the manometer at a point approximately level with the right atrium of the patient's heart (see photos 1 and 2). That is a

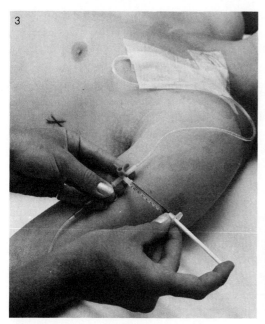

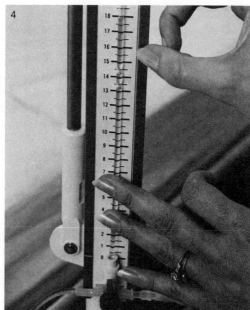

midaxillary line measuring about 10-12 cm from the posterior surface of the patient's body in the fourth intercostal space.

• *Reading.* Briefly open the I.V. line completely to make sure it's patent. (If the tubing has run dry or is obstructed, you may have to gently irrigate the line through the stopcock with 1 to 2 cc of sterile normal saline, as shown in photo 3. If the saline won't flow freely into the line, suspect a clot. Flushing with a heparin solution won't dissolve the clot. So, stop the procedure and call the doctor.)

Once you've cleared the I.V. line, turn the manometer stopcock so the solution from the I.V. flows into the manometer until the level reaches about 30 cm. Don't run more solution in; too much may prevent the column from fluctuating or could cause an infection. Close off the I.V. solution by turning the handle of the stopcock toward the I.V. bottle. The solution will now flow from the manometer into the patient. The fluid will drop rapidly down the tube and then come to rest, although it will oscillate by 1-2 cm when the patient breathes. Since air bubbles in the manometer column can skew a reading, eliminate them by flicking the manometer with your finger (photo 4).

• *Determining the level.* The usual CVP reading takes the

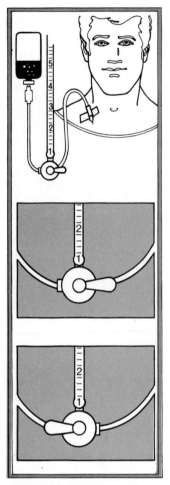

One good turn, then another
Basically, a CVP set-up requires a bottle of I.V. solution, a manometer connected to a three-way stopcock and the catheter (see illustration at top). To fill the manometer, turn the stopcock to the patient (see center illustration). Then, to take a reading, turn the stopcock toward the I.V. tubing (see bottom illustration).

highest point of oscillation. For example, if the solution oscillates between 6 and 7 cm, the CVP reading is 7 cm of water. Or you may record the exact oscillation: "6 to 7 cm water."

After taking the reading, turn the stopcock to close the manometer line. Once again, the solution will flow from the I.V. bottle into the patient.

After recording the reading, apply an occlusive dressing over the catheter at the point of insertion. Write the date and time on a piece of adhesive tape applied over the dressing itself, so that other staff members will know when it should be changed. Generally, CVP dressings are changed every 72 hours.

• *Recognizing false results.* Take every precaution to avoid a false reading. False high readings can be caused by restless patients changing position, simultaneous use of a respirator for the patient, clots obstructing the CVP line, or incorrect leveling of the manometer. False high or low readings can be caused by an inaccurately placed catheter. (Only an X-ray can reliably indicate the catheter's position.)

What does it mean?
CVP readings normally range from 5 to 15 cm. The reading reflects the quantity of circulating blood (blood volume), the efficiency of the heart as a pump (cardiac function), and the contraction or relaxation of the blood vessels (vascular tone). If the reading is abnormal, a change has occurred in one or more of these. If, for example, cardiac function is stable, an abnormal CVP level will indicate alterations in either blood volume, vascular tone, or both. If the cardiac function and vascular tone are stable, the abnormal level will indicate changes in blood volume. Similarly, if vascular tone and blood volume are stable, variations will indicate a change in cardiac function.

So, an elevated reading (over 15 cm) may be a sign of vasoconstriction, right ventricular failure secondary to left heart failure, cardiac tamponade, hypertension, hypervolemia caused by infusion overload, ascites compressing the vena cava, valvular stenosis, or heart compression caused by a rigid pericardial membrane. A low reading (below 5 cm) may be a sign of vasodilation, peripheral blood pooling, hypovolemia, rapid ascites, or angioneurotic edema.

But other conditions also can cause CVP measurements to

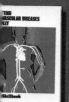
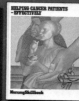
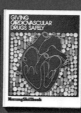
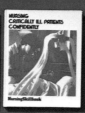
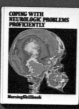
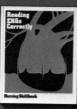
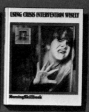

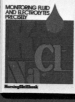
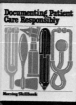
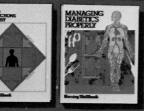
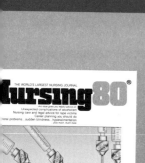

Choose one of these important books as your introductory volume when you join the **NURSING SKILLBOOK** series...the most comprehensive reference series ever published for nurses.

• Using Crisis Intervention Wisely • Coping With Neurologic Problems Proficiently • Managing Diabetics Properly • Helping Cancer Patients Effectively • Documenting Patient Care Responsibly • Monitoring Fluid and Electrolytes Precisely • Giving Cardiovascular Drugs Safely • Assessing Vital Functions Accurately • Nursing Critically Ill Patients Confidently • Giving Emergency Care Competently • Reading EKGs Correctly • Combatting Cardiovascular Diseases Skillfully • Dealing with Death and Dying

BUSINESS REPLY MAIL
FIRST CLASS PERMIT NO. 1903 HICKSVILLE, N.Y.

POSTAGE WILL BE PAID BY ADDRESSEE

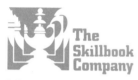

The
Skillbook
Company

6 Commercial Street
Hicksville, N.Y. 11801

BUSINESS REPLY MAIL
FIRST CLASS PERMIT NO. 217 MARION, OHIO

POSTAGE WILL BE PAID BY ADDRESSEE

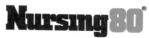

P.O. Box 3744
One Health Road
Marion, Ohio 43302

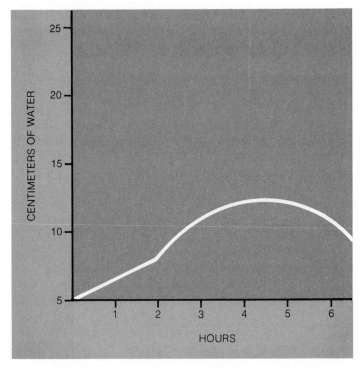

On the right track
To track the heart's ongoing ability to handle returned blood, you must take CVP readings at regular intervals. Eventually these readings will form a curve. This curve, for instance, shows readings taken at 1-hour intervals after administration of 2 units of blood.

vary: urinary output, arterial blood pressure, respiratory rate, emotional state, parenteral administration of fluids, tension pneumothorax, and massive hemothorax. Obviously, then, one single reading is of restricted value, for it merely indicates the heart's competency to handle returned blood at that time. So, you must take a series of readings — spaced at intervals of 15, 30, or 60 minutes apart. And you must correlate each additional reading with previous ones, and with data from other observations. For example, you can evaluate vascular stability by skin temperature, tone, and color, and by capillary and venous filling times. Take these findings into account, as well as those indicating respiratory and heart rates. Over a period of time, a CVP curve will be established (see diagram).

How well does it work?
The practical clinical value of the CVP can perhaps be best illustrated by the following case.

A patient who had had a mitral valve replacement began hemorrhaging 2 hours postop. He was taken back to surgery

Sidestepping potential perils
Dangers of CVP monitoring
include possible air embolus or
hemorrhage caused by a
disconnected or broken catheter;
thromboembolism caused by
clots in the CVP line; and local or
systemic infection caused by
long-term use or careless
handling of the catheter, I.V.
solutions, or I.V. tubing. To avoid
these dangers, secure all tubing
connections with ½ inch tape;
add 500-1000 units of heparin to
I.V. solution or flush with small
(usually 2 cc) boluses of
heparinized solution; and change
dressings every 72 hours.

for resuturing. When he returned to the floor, he showed all the signs of hypovolemic shock: cold and moist skin, alertness with restlessness, collapse of peripheral veins, and an arterial systolic pressure of 80-90 mm Hg.

The nurse took a CVP reading to test her suspicions; it read 1 to 2 cm — a clear confirmation of hypovolemia. On the doctor's order, she gave the patient 1 unit of blood in 15 minutes; his CVP climbed to 5 cm. She gave another unit; his CVP climbed to 10 cm. After a third transfusion, his CVP reached 15 cm — normal for that patient.

In this case, the nurse used the CVP to test her suspicion of hypovolemic shock. If the reading had been as high as 10 or 15 cm, she would have known that his blood volume was adequate — and then would have gone on to test his cardiac function, respiratory status, and vascular tone.

In all such cases, your role in monitoring central venous pressure consists of observing carefully, evaluating what you've observed, and taking appropriate action. To do all this, you must know the proper method for obtaining a reading. By knowing the patient's cardiac competence and general vascular tone, you then can give appropriate — maybe even life-saving — nursing care.

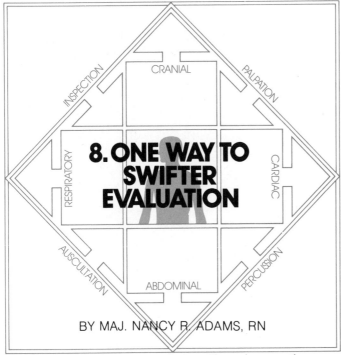

8. ONE WAY TO SWIFTER EVALUATION

BY MAJ. NANCY R. ADAMS, RN

HELPFUL AS THE CENTRAL venous catheter is, sometimes you may be called upon to monitor a patient's cardiac status with another cardiac catheter — the Swan-Ganz catheter. In fact, this catheter is becoming the analyzer of choice in many ICUs, CCUs, and even medical units. Why? Quite simply because it overcomes the limitations of the central venous catheter.

First, the central venous catheter doesn't always reveal dysfunction promptly enough. Sometimes, in fact, a patient has all the clinical signs of left ventricular failure and pulmonary congestion, yet the CVP still reads normal. The Swan-Ganz catheter on the other hand, can detect changes in cardiac performance and the vascular system before overt complications, such as rales or pulmonary edema, appear.

Second, the CVP doesn't correlate with left ventricular end diastolic pressure (LVEDP) in patients with hepatic failure, peritonitis, multiple trauma, or left ventricular dysfunction following myocardial infarction. Readings from the Swan-Ganz catheter do.

Finally, CVP readings fluctuate with changes in the venous tone and compliance of the right ventricle. CVP readings reliably measure right heart function, systemic venous com-

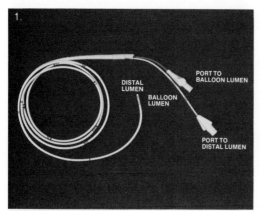

Double lumen catheter

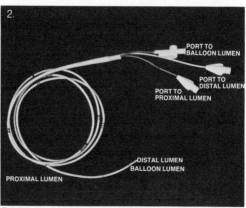

Triple lumen catheter

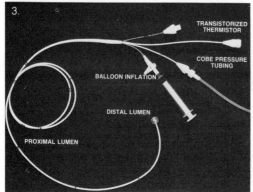

Thermodilution catheter

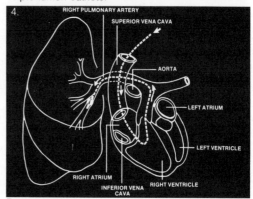

Route of insertion

The simplest type of Swan-Ganz catheter is the double lumen catheter (1). One of its lumens is used to inflate the catheter's balloon, located 1 mm from the catheter tip. When inflated in a peripheral pulmonary vessel, the balloon occludes a portion of the vessel. The second lumen, at the catheter tip, then measures pressure in front of the balloon. This lumen can be used to monitor PAP and PWP, to sample mixed venous blood, and to infuse intravenous solutions.

The second type of Swan-Ganz catheter, known as the triple lumen catheter (2), has an additional, proximal lumen located 30 cm from the catheter tip. When the tip of the catheter rests in the main pulmonary artery, the proximal lumen lies in the right atrium. It may be used to administer fluid or, with the attachment of a transducer, to monitor right atrial pressure (CVP).

The third type, the thermodilution catheter (3), also has a transistorized thermistor to detect changes in blood temperature. Blood temperatures are then used to compute cardiac output.

A physician must insert a Swan-Ganz catheter, usually at the patient's bedside. He inserts it through a peripheral vein, usually the antecubital or subclavian, using a cutdown incision or a percutaneous needle introducer. Then he threads it through the vein to the right atrium, through the right ventricle, and out to the pulmonary artery (see figure 4). Inflation of the balloon propels the catheter through the heart without damaging the ventricle walls.

Once the catheter is in place and the balloon has been deflated, it's no more bothersome to the patient than an ordinary intravenous line.

pliance, and intravascular volume *only* if the patient has no significant cardiopulmonary disease. The Swan-Ganz catheter measures them even if the patient has cardiopulmonary disease.

But don't let these stellar benefits blind you to the complexity of the Swan-Ganz catheter. To make it a safe analyzer, you must know how to get accurate readings.

When inserted in the pulmonary artery, the Swan-Ganz catheter indicates left ventricular filling pressure by measuring pulmonary artery pressure (PAP) and pulmonary wedge pressure (PWP). (At the end of the diastolic phase — before the next systolic contraction occurs — the left ventricle, left atrium, and pulmonary vascular bed momentarily act as a single chamber. So, changes in the left side of the heart appear in the PAP and PWP.)

Taking a pressure reading

After the doctor has inserted the catheter, inflate the balloon to take a reading. Ideally you should use carbon dioxide to inflate it, since CO_2 is 20 times more blood-soluble than air — an advantage if the balloon ruptures. But most hospitals routinely inflate with air. (Never use air for inflation if the balloon could enter arterial circulation, however, as in a patient with a suspected right-to-left intracardiac shunt or a pulmonary arteriovenous shunt. Although 1 to 2 cc of air in venous circulation won't harm a patient, the same amount in arterial circulation can harm him.)

Never use normal saline or another liquid for inflation. The viscosity and capillary action of fluids prevent the balloon from completely deflating. Also, a fluid-filled balloon impairs the flow-directed sensitivity of the catheter.

Inflate carefully. The balloon is quite fragile and, even with the most meticulous care, may disintegrate 48 hours after insertion.

Before inflating the balloon for a pressure reading, flush the entire line. You may flush it manually by injecting 3 to 5 cc of heparinized solution (1000 units heparin in 250 cc normal saline). Or, you may keep an I.V. infusion with 4000 units heparin per liter running at an open rate (10 cc per hour); you may keep a regular I.V. flow going with 20 cc per hour with 1000 units heparin added to each liter; you may provide a continuous irrigation of 3 to 4 cc per hour with the Sorenson

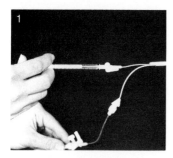

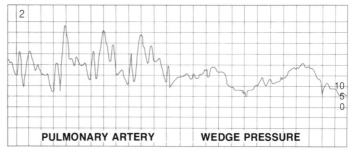

PULMONARY ARTERY   WEDGE PRESSURE

PAP, PWP, and output
No matter what kind of catheter you use, you'll have to inflate the balloon as shown above to get a reading. Look for the tracing to change from PAP to PWP (see diagram above) and compare readings with the norms shown on the facing page. If you're using a thermodilution catheter, the doctor may also want you to measure cardiac output, as shown in the pictures on page 105.

Valve; or you may use a bolus irrigation when the Sorenson Valve is open by pulling the rubber tail.

1. Make sure the balloon is completely deflated. Then, inflate the balloon with the smallest syringe (T.B.) that will give the required amount of air. A size 7 French catheter requires no more than 1.5 ml of air; a size 5 French catheter requires no more than 0.8 ml. (I don't recommend use of the side arm to close off the balloon lumen. It doesn't give you a quick way of identifying whether the balloon has deflated completely. Also, the arm can break from frequent manipulation.)

2. Inflate slowly. Stop inflating when the pressure curve changes from pulmonary to wedge pressure. Overdistention could produce pulmonary vessel damage or balloon rupture.

Avoid lengthy balloon inflations for wedge readings. Since the inflated balloon occludes a portion of the pulmonary artery, prolonged inflation could produce a local infarction.

If the syringe plunger doesn't spring back when you release it, suspect balloon rupture. Don't try to inflate the balloon again; that would cause air emboli in the venous circulation.

After the pressure reading, flush the entire line again. Reposition the Palley Manifold or stopcock to open the flow of the heparinized solution to the patient.

What do the readings mean?
The graphs on the opposite page show normal pressures.

An increase in PWP indicates an increase in LVEDP. And a markedly high LVEDP indicates left ventricular dysfunction, which causes decreased cardiac output.

A decrease in PWP, on the other hand, indicates a decrease in LVEDP. And a low LVEDP also indicates decreased cardiac output.

Generally, an acute rise in the PAP while the PWP remains normal suggests a primary pulmonary disorder, such as a

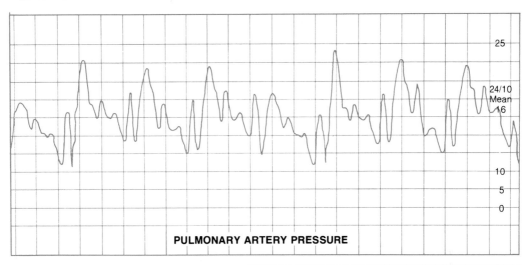

PULMONARY ARTERY PRESSURE

25

24/10
Mean
16

10
5
0

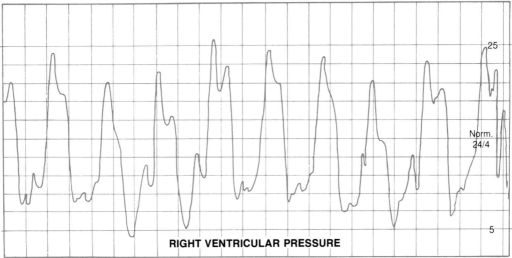

RIGHT VENTRICULAR PRESSURE

25

Norm.
24/4

5

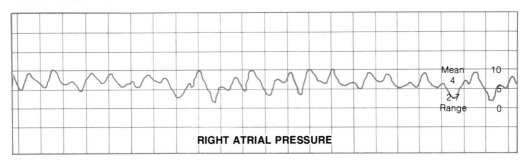

RIGHT ATRIAL PRESSURE

Mean
4

2-7
Range

10
5
0

pulmonary embolism. An increase in both PAP and PWP suggests a primary cardiac problem, such as left ventricular failure.

Remember, though, that PWP readings aren't absolutes. At some point, PWP and LVEDP readings diverge, although physicians disagree over where that point is. Also, mitral-valve obstruction can upset the correlation between PWP and LVEDP.

Optimum wedge pressure readings also vary according to each patient's condition. Patients who've had acute myocardial infarction that altered their left ventricular filling pressure should have pressures maintained at 14 to 18 mm Hg. (Pressures below 14 mm Hg reduce ventricular performance; pressures above 18 mm Hg cause pulmonary congestion.)

Positive end expiratory pressure (PEEP) also may interfere with PWP readings and their correlation to left atrial pressure and LVEDP. Although small amounts of PEEP (less than 5 cm) won't affect readings, larger amounts (5 to 15 cm) may increase the PWP by inhibiting venous return from the pulmonary vasculature and by causing pulmonary congestion. Cardiac output will fall as a result. To determine whether PEEP is inhibiting cardiac output, take pressure readings while patients are on the ventilator. If it is, the physician may elect to reduce the PEEP.

Throughout insertion, keep a careful watch on the pressure tracings for signs of other problems. Absence of a PWP tracing usually indicates rupture of the balloon. Absence of *all* pressure tracings indicates a faulty transducer or, more likely, a clot in the distal lumen. (To avoid dislodging a clot into the pulmonary circulation, try to aspirate it before irrigating the lumen.)

After insertion, watch for other problems that may arise from changes in the catheter's position. If a constant wedge-pressure tracing appears on the oscilloscope and you can't obtain a higher amplitude PAP, the catheter is probably stranded in the wedge position. Notify the physician immediately so he can pull back the catheter before it causes a local pulmonary artery infarct.

Inability to obtain a wedge pressure may be due to a balloon rupture or slipping of the catheter back into the right ventricle. If the catheter has slipped out of position, it will show up on an X-ray; if the balloon has ruptured, air injected into the catheter won't encounter any resistance. (After a balloon rupture, you won't be able to obtain any reading but a PAP. But, unless the patient has a primary problem with an increase in pulmonary vascular resistance, the PAP will give a fairly reliable indication of left atrial pressure.)

Damping of the pressure tracing may be an early sign of partial obstruction of the lumen. Try to aspirate the obstruction and then clear the line with a bolus irrigation of saline. Also, change the position of the patient's arm; this may increase the amplitude of the tracing.

Measuring other indices

Sometimes you'll need to measure other indices of cardiac function, such as cardiac output or mixed venous oxygen tension.

If you're using a thermodilution catheter, you'll need a thermodilution cardiac output computer to measure cardiac output. When programmed with figures for body temperature and cooled injectate temperature, the computer measures the change in pulmonary artery blood temperature registered by the thermistor at the catheter tip. From this, it determines output in liters per minute. Normal cardiac output for an average adult is 5 to 6 liters per minute, or 2.8 to 4.2 liters per minute per square meter of body surface area.

3. After the doctor has inserted the thermodilution catheter, connect it to the cardiac output computer.

4. Fill a large basin with normal saline and a large quantity of ice. Place two bottles of the dextrose in water in the basin; leave one bottle capped and place a Centigrade thermometer in the other. (You may fit the thermometer through the rubber stopper, or you may remove the rubber stopper completely.) The bottle with the thermometer serves as a control to determine the temperature of the solution in the other bottle, which you will use for the actual injection.

5. When the thermometer registers 0° C., usually 30 minutes after you place the bottle in the ice, the injection solution is ready. (You can hasten the chilling process by storing bottles of injection solution in the refrigerator.) Draw up 10 cc of the solution. Take the patient's temperature and record it.

6. Then, inject the 10 cc of chilled solution into the proximal lumen over a period of 2 to 3 seconds. Make sure the stopcock is off to the Sorenson Valve during this procedure.

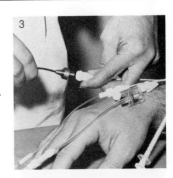

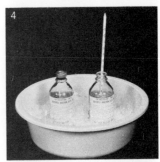

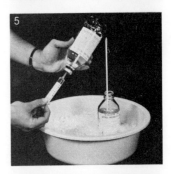

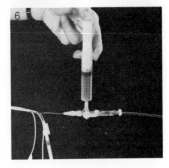

Be sure you don't inject the chilled solution too slowly. If you do, the signal peak may be too low to register, resulting in an erroneously high or nonreproducible cardiac output. Also be sure the patient doesn't hyperventilate or breathe heavily during this procedure; that will cause the pulmonary artery temperature to vary and produce an unstable thermal baseline. Finally, make sure the catheter isn't wedged during injection. If it is, only a portion of the chilled solution will reach the catheter tip and you'll get a falsely high reading.

Watch the computer for the cardiac output computation. Do at least three computations.

Occasionally you also may withdraw mixed venous blood directly from the pulmonary artery to measure mixed venous oxygen tension (normal: about 40 mm Hg), which indicates the adequacy of intracellular oxygenation, and send for analysis to determine the degree of pulmonary shunting. Withdraw blood through the distal stopcock, being sure to keep it sterile. After withdrawing the blood, flush the line thoroughly to prevent clogging. (If you can't administer medications any other way, you also can inject them through the proximal lumen.)

With all of these readings, you'll have a clear picture of your patient's cardiac status.

SKILLCHECK 3

1. John Freed, a 49-year-old executive, was admitted to your unit with an extensive anterior wall MI. During the first 24 hours, his vital signs remained stable and routine CVP ranged between 8 and 10 cm H_2O. Now, on the third day, his CVP has risen to 14 cm H_2O and his pulse rate has increased slightly from 90 to 100.

What would you suspect? What assessments would you make?

2. Last evening, Marvin Kohn was admitted with crushing chest pain. On admission, he had crepitant rales in both lung bases, an S_3, and positive hepato-jugular reflex. An EKG revealed ST elevation in leads V_1-V_3, poor progression of precordial R waves, and reciprocal changes of ST depression in the opposite leads (inferior-lateral). The doctor placed him on furosemide (Lasix) 80 mg Stat, isosorbide dinitrate (Isordil), 20 mg q.i.d., and chlordiazepoxide hydrochloride (Librium), 10 mg q.i.d.

Today your examination reveals persistent rales, a somewhat louder S_3, and II/VI holosystolic murmur at the mitral valve. Mr. Kohn's vital signs are stable, his intake 1000 cc, and his output 600 cc.

What would you suspect is happening to Mr. Kohn? What nursing assessments should you make?

3. Karen Porter, a 58-year-old housewife, came to the CCU with sudden anterior nonradiating chest pain. Serial EKGs and enzymes revealed an inferior wall myocardial infarction.

Mrs. Porter's vital signs remained stable: blood pressure, 130/80; pulse, 90; and respirations, 22. The doctor routinely inserted a CVP, and readings held steady at 10-14 cm H_2O. Her intake and output were normal, and her EKG showed normal sinus rhythm. She had no S_3 or S_4 rales, and p.r.n. nitroglycerin relieved her occasional chest pains. After an uncomplicated hospital stay of 2 weeks, Mrs. Porter was discharged.

What assessment would you have made for Mrs. Porter during her hospitalization?

4. Mr. Barker, a 49-year-old executive, was admitted to the CCU with severe, sharp, radiating chest pain. Vital signs on admission were: pulse, 100-110; temperature, 99° F; respiration, 24 regular; blood pressure, 150/80 to 160/90. An EKG revealed sinus tachycardia with ST elevation in leads V_2-V_6 and reciprocal ST depression in L_2-L_3 and aVF.

On doctor's orders, you place Mr. Barker on complete bedrest with an I.V. of D_5W, nitroglycerin p.r.n. for chest pain, P.O. diazepam (Valium) p.r.n. for sedation, propranolol (Inderal) 10 mg P.O. q.i.d., and Isordil 5 mg every four hours. For the first three days after admission, Mr. Barker seems to be doing well; his vital signs remain stable. But suddenly his blood pressure drops to 130/80, then to 88/68. Serial enzymes are elevated, his heart rate has increased to 120-130 sinus tachycardia, and his respirations have fallen to 30-32, dyspneic. His input/output ratio also has fallen from 1200/1000 to 1400/600 — less than 30 cc/hr output.

When you auscultate, you find bilateral rales from base to scapula, and an S_3 ventricular gallop rhythm. The doctor orders O_2 therapy at 5 L/min via nasal catheter and inserts a Swan-Ganz catheter antecubitally. An X-ray reveals an enlarged heart with signs of interstitial edema; PAP is 50 cm H_2O and PWP is 20 cm H_2O.

What do you think is happening to Mr. Barker? What assessments should you make?

5. Pat Sell, 29 years old, has been hospitalized with heart failure resulting from congenital aortic stenosis. Early assessments reveal severe dyspnea, elevated heart rate, fatigue, and sinus tachycardia. Her blood pressure at admission seems relatively stable. The doctor starts her on I.V. fluids and I.V. furosemide (Lasix). Diuresis is excellent and Pat rapidly improves — until the sixth day.

On the sixth day, Pat's heart rate climbs again, this time to 140, and she complains of fatigue and dyspnea. The doctor orders continuation of the previous treatment, with the addition of maintenance P.O. digoxin.

What assessments would be most important?

(answers on page 183)

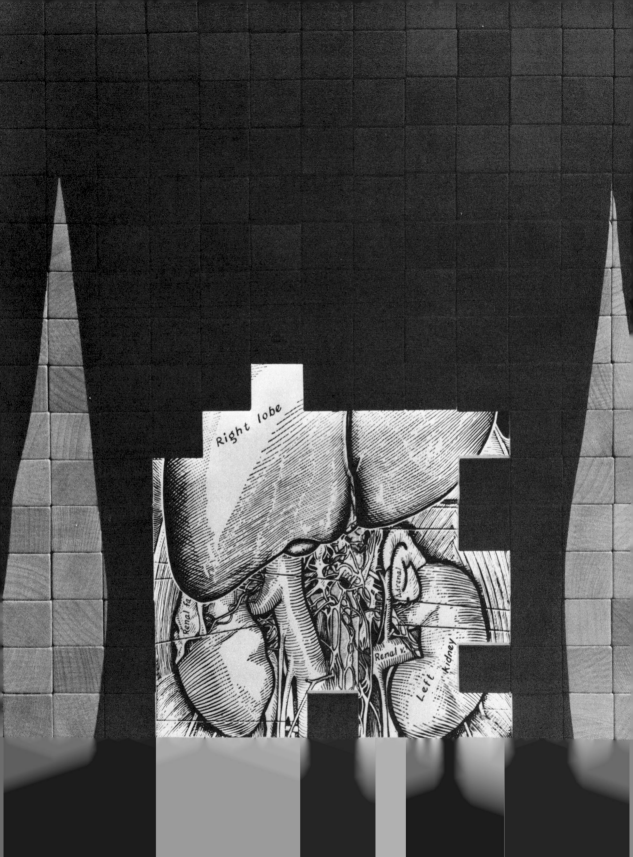

ASSESSING ABDOMINAL ORGAN FUNCTION

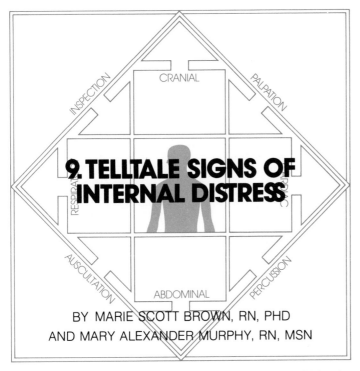

9. TELLTALE SIGNS OF INTERNAL DISTRESS

INSPECTION CRANIAL PALPATION RESPIRATORY AUSCULTATION ABDOMINAL PERCUSSION

BY MARIE SCOTT BROWN, RN, PHD
AND MARY ALEXANDER MURPHY, RN, MSN

MANY OF THE BODY'S vital processes take place within the abdomen. Just think of it: This great bony bowl of rib, spine, and pelvis houses much of digestion, assimilation, excretion, and hormonal regulation. Yet assessing these functions without sophisticated equipment can be far trickier than assessing respiratory or cardiac function. After all, when assessing respiratory or cardiac function you can rely on obvious norms, such as respiratory or pulse rate. But when assessing organs such as the liver or GI tract, you don't have such norms to rely on. So, you have to depend on your overall assessment of the abdomen...and your ability to pick up telltale signs of malfunction.

In exploring the abdomen from without, you'll use all four methods of examination. But you had best follow inspection with auscultation (instead of the usual order of percussion or palpation) because either percussion or palpation can easily disturb the normal sounds.

You can subdivide the abdomen to examine it by either of two accepted methods. The traditional method somewhat laboriously divides it into nine sections. More popular today, and the one we use, is the simpler method of dividing the

To divide and conquer
This figure illustrates two systems
for describing the abdomen: The
older method divides it into nine
segments, the newer into
quadrants. You can identify the
organs in each quadrant by
percussing and palpating.

LEFT UPPER
QUADRANT
Left lobe of liver
Spleen
Stomach
Left kidney
Body and tail of
  pancreas
Splenic flexure of
  colon

LEFT LOWER
QUADRANT
Sigmoid colon
Left uterine tube
Left ovary
Left ureter

RIGHT UPPER
QUADRANT
Right lobe of liver
Gallbladder
Pylorus
Duodenum
Head of the
  pancreas
Upper part of
  right kidney
Hepatic flexure of
  colon

RIGHT LOWER
QUADRANT
Lower portion of
  right kidney
Cecum
Appendix
Ascending colon
Right uterine tube
Right ovary
Right ureter

MIDLINE
Uterus
Urinary bladder

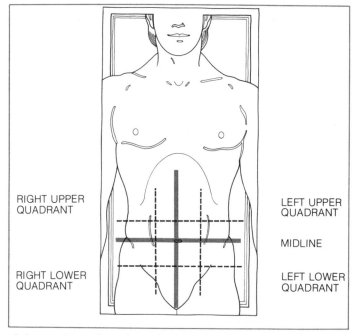

abdomen by a line through the middle, both vertically and
horizontally, into quadrants, as shown in the accompanying
drawing. The only instrument you will need to help you in your
examinaton is the stethoscope.

Tenderness, masses, and organomegaly are the signs to look
out for when you examine the abdomen.

Inspection
Look first for movement. Normally you should see only the
movement of breathing. Any adult using his abdominal muscles to breathe should be carefully checked for thoracic problems.

You don't normally see peristalsis. If you do see peristaltic
waves, it can mean a gastrointestinal obstruction. Reverse
peristaltic waves can be found with malrotation of the bowel,
duodenal ulcer, duodenal stenosis, gastrointestinal allergy, or
even urinary tract infection.

Contour also can tell you something. The abdomen normally bulges a little at the beginning of inspiration. But with
certain central nervous system diseases such as chorea it may
retract rather than bulge: This paradoxical inspiration is called

Czerny's sign. Note any localized fullness, too. If you find it in the right lower quadrant, it may be an appendiceal abscess.

A potbelly may be normal in obese patients. Nonetheless you should investigate it, for it may conceal organomegaly, ascites, neoplasm, cyst, or some defect in the abdominal wall.

Severe abdominal distention may indicate starvation. But a lesser degree of distention may mean fecal retention (in megacolon, the masses will feel plastic), organomegaly, or, in a woman, ovarian cysts or pregnancy.

Bulging of the flanks may indicate ascites, which often accompanies liver disease such as cirrhosis. If you suspect ascites, look for glistening thick skin; it can indicate ascites or underlying edema.

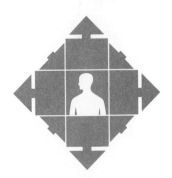

Health history:
What you should know
1. Does the patient have a history of abdominal illness? Has he undergone surgery?
2. What is his diet? Does he take medication? Does he use a prosthesis?
3. Does he suffer from pain, nausea, vomiting, weight gain or loss, digestive problems?

Superficial vessels should also be observed in the abdomen. In thin patients you can sometimes see a pulsating aorta over the epigastrium. But excess pulsation radiating equally in all directions may indicate an aortic aneurysm. And excess pulsation spreading only in an anterior direction may indicate a tumor over the aorta. Dilated veins may indicate partial obstruction of the vascular system. If you want to check vascular obstruction, remember that the pattern of venous filling radiates from the umbilicus: Above it, veins refill from the bottom up; below the umbilicus they fill from the top down. Obstruction of the inferior vena cava can result in reversed filling below the umbilicus, whereas reversed filling above it may mean obstruction of the superior vena cava.

Hair distribution can be significant. Hairiness may be familial, or a sign of adrenocortical problems. You can expect to find a triangular pubic hair pattern in women, a diamond-shaped one in men. Although variations from this pattern may be normal, they may indicate endocrine or liver disorders. A diamond-shaped pattern in a woman, for instance, may indicate a tumor of the adrenal gland; a triangular pattern in a man may indicate cirrhosis.

A bluish umbilicus — Cullen's sign — may occur with intra-abdominal hemorrhage; a nodular one — Sister Joseph's nodule — may signify abdominal cancer. If the umbilicus is everted without hernia, it may be from some kind of increased intra-abdominal pressure.

Auscultation
The first sound to assess is that of peristalsis. If you don't hear

it at once, don't conclude it doesn't exist; peristaltic sounds can be so irregular that you'll have to listen at least 5 minutes by the clock. Paralytic ileus is unusual in ambulatory patients; when it does exist it most often comes from diffuse peritoneal irritation. Hyperperistalsis occurs with diarrhea, and more severely with early obstruction in the intestine or pylorus. This is a frequent high-pitched tinkling accompanied by pain.

Listen for vascular sounds, too. Venous hums like those sometimes heard in the neck may accompany abnormalities of the umbilical vein, vascular problems of the portal system, or hemangiomas of the liver. A murmur near the umbilicus may mean a renal artery defect. Friction rubs are sometimes detectable in the abdomen. They may originate in an inflamed spleen or tumorous liver, or with generalized peritoneal obstruction. These rubs can be so soft as to be taken for breath sounds.

A bruit, similar to a murmur, is important only if you hear it despite change of position and with the stethoscope held very lightly against the abdominal wall. Then it may signify a vascular problem — a dilated, tortuous, or constricted vessel; if over the aorta, it could be a sign of aneurysm or, in some other place, of congenital bands elsewhere in the vascular system.

You also can hear stomach contents. To do this, hold the stethoscope high on the stomach and rock the patient back and forth. If the stomach contains the normal amount of fluid, you'll hear a splash.

Percussion
Stand at the patient's right side and begin on the left thorax, going down the midaxillary line. You should encounter a tympanitic or drumlike note where the lung overlies the splenic flexure at the head of the descending colon. Above the ninth rib interspace, dullness may originate with the spleen. Occasionally, though, this note may be produced by a kidney, the left lobe of the liver, or even consolidation of the left lower lung.

From the left side, repeat the percussion down the right midaxillary line. You can expect to find liver dullness at the sixth rib or interspace anteriorly, the ninth rib posteriorly. But there may be relative dullness one or two interspaces above this. You should encounter the lower border of the liver at the costal margin.

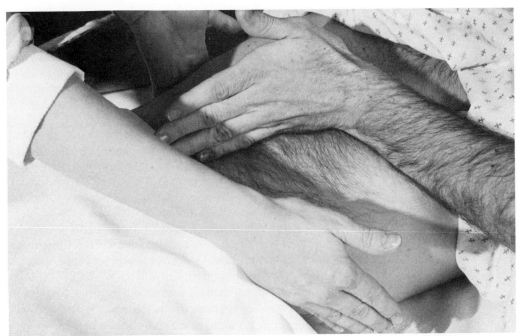

The liver moves with respiration, so if you percuss it during inspiration, and then during held expiration, it should move about two fingerbreadths. The rest of the abdomen should be tympanitic. But it may be unusually so in patients who habitually swallow air (such as patients with laryngectomies) or in those with an obstructive lesion of the GI tract.

Shifting dullness can indicate ascites. You will hear dullness in the midabdomen when the patient is standing, but when he is lying on his back the dullness will shift to his flanks. If you roll him on his side, it will shift to the dependent side.

The wave of ascites
Inspect the patient for symmetrical distention of the abdomen. If you suspect ascites, perform the fluid-wave test: Place the patient's hand in his midline to prevent transmission of the wave through the abdominal wall. Holding your left hand against his right side, strike his left side with the pad of your palm. If the patient has ascites, you will feel a sharp slap against your left hand as the wave is transmitted through the fluid.

Palpation
Use a light touch. And for goodness' sake, have your hands warm: Cold fingers can make for such muscular contraction that you'll learn little. Flexing the patient's knees and putting a pillow under his head may take strain off the abdominal muscles and lessen the resistance to your probing.

Begin with superficial palpation, and gradually increase the pressure. You can feel certain types of masses such as a cyst or hematoma of the rectus muscles this way. You may also encounter the rebound tenderness of Blumberg's sign in which

**Here you feel it,
there you don't**
Most internal organs have no pain receptors. Visceral pain, however, may be referred; that is, the patient may feel pain far from its actual source. (See illustration on opposite page.) One possible explanation for this phenomenon is that neurons from the affected organ enter the same spinal cord segment as do neurons from the area where the pain is felt. Impulses from these neurons become confused when they reach the brain. Gallbladder pain, for example, frequently radiates from the epigastrium to the scapular region.

a pain occurs when you abruptly release pressure over McBurney's point, thus indicating peritoneal inflammation.

If you feel freely movable, nontender bubbles directly under the skin, it is subcutaneous crepitus. It may indicate subcutaneous emphysema or gas gangrene. You can also evaluate muscle tone through palpation. Involuntary abdominal muscle rigidity on one or both sides can be an important sign of peritoneal irritation.

After the entire abdomen has been superficially palpated, perform deep palpation over the same area. Deep palpation is important for discovering masses, tenderness, deep vessels, and palpable organs. An important clue here is tenderness. Remember, though, that the last area to be palpated is the area in which you suspect any pathology.

Some pain, like that originating in the appendix, which can hurt almost anywhere in the abdomen before settling in the right lower quadrant, will start out poorly localized and then gradually become more definite.

It is normal to complain of pain or wince during deep palpation of the midepigastrium; this is the area of the aorta. But other areas of pain should be carefully noted. Remember, pain is often referred by certain pathways to other locations.

• Pain originating in the common bile duct may be referred to the epigastrium and may radiate to the right scapular region.

• Pain in the kidneys, ovaries, fallopian tubes, or ureters may be felt in the ipsilateral flank.

• Splenic pain may be referred to the left shoulder.

Remember, too, that:

• Rebound pain occurs only if the peritoneum is involved; this occurs even when pressure is exerted far from the diseased area, and may come from coughing or straining.

• Pain caused by inflammation is generally *constant,* or even increases, when pressure is applied.

• Visceral pain caused by distention or contraction of an organ *lessens* under constant pressure.

Deep palpation
Besides abdominal tenderness, deep palpation can reveal masses, deep vessels, and palpable organs. Evaluate all masses for their size, consistency, tenderness, mobility, position, shape, pulsatility, and surface characteristics. But if there is any question of neoplasm, be careful. Excess manipulation may spread it.

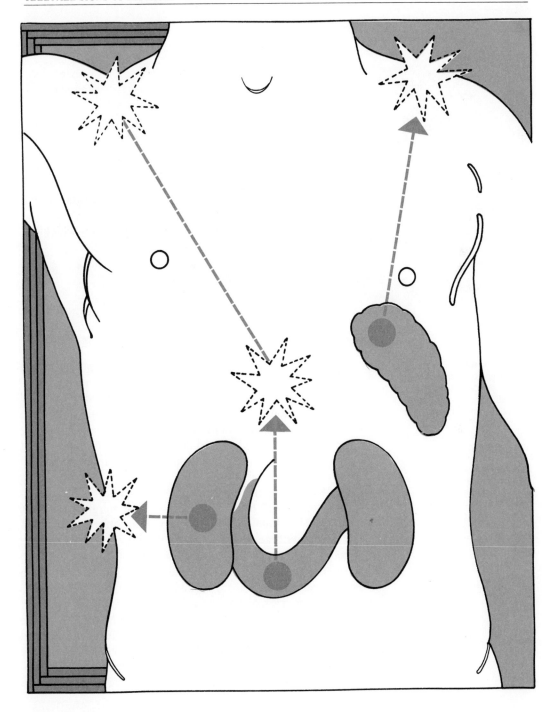

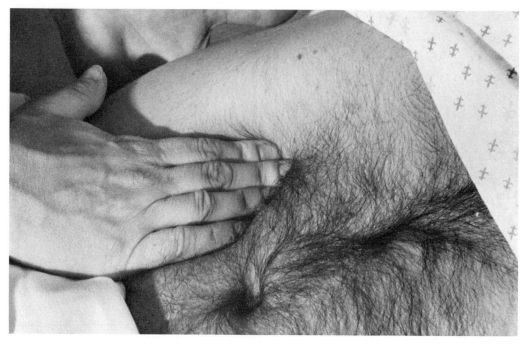

The liver's edge
Usually you can feel the liver edge at the right costal margin. Place your left hand behind, parallel to, and supporting the eleventh and twelfth ribs. Press up. Press your right hand gently but deeply below the right costal margin. Have the patient take a deep breath; you may feel the firm, smooth liver edge tap your fingers. If it seems enlarged, note how many centimeters it extends below the costal margin.

You can sometimes palpate fecal masses in patients with constipation. If they seem excessive, check for megacolon.

Some vessels can be felt with deep palpation. Femoral pulses are among them, although these will sometimes have been encountered with superficial palpation. You can usually palpate the aorta, and should do so carefully to make sure it doesn't balloon out in width, which may spell aneurysm.

Liver: Evaluating the edge
If the liver doesn't extend below the costal margin, you can't feel it. But by palpating with the flat of your fingers, starting at the lower abdomen and gradually working higher, you may touch the liver edge. If so, note the feel: A firm, sharp edge is normal; a blunt edge may indicate passive congestion; and a nodular edge may indicate portal cirrhosis. If the liver extends below the costal margin, it may be enlarged; consult a doctor.

In rare instances of congenital anomaly called Riedel's lobe (associated with chronic gallstones) the liver will extend downward on the right side. Sometimes you can feel systolic pulsations in the liver of a patient with certain cardiac problems. That situation calls for referral. A tender liver may

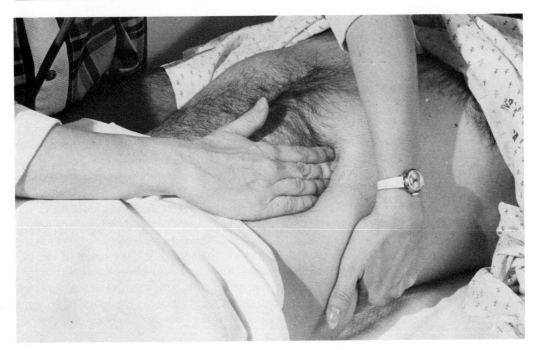

indicate infectious hepatitis, mononucleosis, liver abscess, or some other acute inflammatory disorder.

Intestines: Palpable in part

Normally you can palpate only two parts of the intestine: the cecum and the sigmoid. The cecum feels like a soft, gas-filled object in the right lower quadrant. The sigmoid feels like a freely movable, sausage-shaped mass, and is normally tender; you can roll it over the pelvic rim in the left lower quadrant. You may be able to feel other parts of the intestine if they're distended, inflamed, obstructed, or tumorous. In chronic ulcerative colitis, for example, the ascending, descending, and sigmoid colons may all be palpable and tender.

Whenever a portion of the intestines is distended with gas and fluid, as with obstruction, it will be palpable and tender. Obstruction of the small bowel will show up as distention of the lower abdomen.

You also can palpate the spleen if it is enlarged. (Normally you can feel the tip.) If you suspect splenomegaly, as with mononucleosis, take great care; you could rupture an inflamed spleen.

Touch the spleen's tip

Stand at the patient's right side with your right hand behind his left costovertebral area and push gently up from behind. With your opposite hand, work gently under the left anterior costal margin. Get the patient to take a deep breath. Because inspiration pushes down on the spleen, the tip should strike your left fingers.

Some clinicians, though, prefer to palpate the spleen by ballottement. To do this, again push frontward gently from behind the costovertebral angle with the right hand; with the left, push against the abdominal wall just under the costal margin in short, ballotting movements. If the spleen is there, you will feel the tip bounce back against the ballotting fingers. You can feel it more easily if the patient rolls over onto his right side.

In palpation, practice will acquaint you soon enough with the abdominal landmarks. Beyond that, experience will give it meaning as you acquire skill in assessing the normal, the harmless variations from the normal, and the features of pathology.

Kidneys: Tough to touch

Very few clinicians say they can routinely feel the kidneys, because they are buried so deeply within the abdominal cavity. But you should at least try to palpate for them. Lying immediately adjacent to the vertebral column, the kidneys descend slightly with inspiration; sometimes this allows you to feel the lower pole, particularly of the right kidney since it is lower. Usually you can palpate the higher left kidney only in thin patients with weak abdominal muscles. Tenderness to renal palpation may indicate acute inflammation of the kidneys. If the patient is obese, you can check for tenderness by tapping the costovertebral area with your fist. If you can't feel the kidneys, you can at least rule out hydronephrosis, congenital polycystic disease of the kidneys, and perinephritic abscess.

You normally can't feel the bladder when it's empty. But when it's full, it will feel like a firm, smooth mass. When excessively distended, as with certain types of central nervous system defects or urethral obstruction, you'll even be able to see it swelling up in the abdomen. If you press on it, the patient will feel an urge to urinate.

Of course, to really assess the kidney and bladder, you also have to assess their productivity. And that is covered in the next chapter.

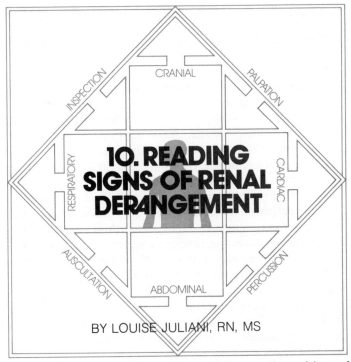

10. READING SIGNS OF RENAL DERANGEMENT

INSPECTION · CRANIAL · PALPATION · RESPIRATORY · CARDIAC · AUSCULTATION · ABDOMINAL · PERCUSSION

BY LOUISE JULIANI, RN, MS

TO KNOW WHAT TO LOOK FOR in examining a patient with renal problems, you have to bear in mind what the kidneys do. These marvelous organs keep constant the body's water, blood solutes, and electrolytes (see NURSING SKILLBOOK *Assessing Fluids and Electrolyte Disorders*). Along with the lungs, they regulate the acid-base balance. They so filter the internal fluids, in fact, that these remain much the same in volume, concentration, and chemical composition despite what is eaten, drunk, taken, excreted, or lost, and notwithstanding the body's other, complicated metabolic processes.

Small wonder, then, that your assessment of renal function is so important, even if it is routine. Simply by noticing the color and smell of urine, for instance, you can detect signs of impending disasters, such as congestive heart failure or renal shutdown. And you can take steps to avert them.

To assess a patient's renal status, you'll have to take his history and observe him for characteristic signs. You'll have to take stock of physical factors that influence the condition of his kidneys. You may have to weigh him each morning for gain or loss of fluid (on the same scale, with the same clothing, after he voids but before he eats). And you'll have to be prepared to

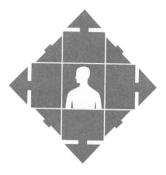

Health history: What you should know
1. Does the patient have diabetes, hypertension, recurrent urinary tract infections, or a history of kidney stones — all of which can point to chronic renal failure?
2. Has he ever worn external drainage equipment?
3. How often does he normally void? Does he have to get up in the night?
4. Does he have any feeling of urgency, any difficulty in starting, or any pain?
5. How much does he void each time — a lot or a little?
6. Is he currently taking diuretics or blood pressure medications?
7. Does he bleed or bruise easily, which can be an early sign of kidney failure?
8. Does he feel restless, sleepless, tired?
9. Does his family have a history of renal problems?

perform a variety of fairly simple diagnostic tests on the unit.

What you see
One of the first things to look for in inspecting this patient is a characteristic change in *pigmentation*. Someone with chronic renal failure is typically pale with a yellow-gray cast to his skin. The pallor comes from erythropoietin-deficiency anemia; the yellow-gray cast, though not clearly understood, may come either from the deposit of a carotene-like substance in the skin or from deranged melanocyte-stimulating hormone — either cause representing a failure of renal excretion.

Many patients in renal failure have dry and itchy skin. They well may have secondary excoriations. And alteration in the clotting mechanism can produce easy bruising or purpura.

The gastrointestinal system is affected by renal problems. Stomatitis can develop, and a urinous breath odor. An early sign of uremia is anorexia, followed by nausea, vomiting, and severe hiccups as the uremia worsens. When you palpate, you may find tenderness in the flank area, as described in the preceding chapter. Or you may find oversized kidneys. You may even feel a kidney tumor.

Hypertension can be a symptom in persons with kidney dysfunction, either as the cause of the kidney problem or as a result of it. Hypertension can stem directly from fluid overload, or it may come from a disruption in the renin-angiotensin system, since renin — an enzyme produced when the kidneys are ischemic — can directly raise the blood pressure. Or the hypertension may result from some unknown cause.

Fluid overload from failing kidneys, when severe enough, can result in congestive heart failure. This comes from expanded blood volume as the result of sodium retention. Many persons with renal failure will experience a sudden change in weight — usually a gain showing frank edema. If you aren't weighing the patient daily, look for periorbital or sacral edema.

The most direct indication of renal function is the quality and quantity of urine. It's a common misconception that the volume of urinary output tells you the state of renal function. But, of course, this isn't true, since failing kidneys can also put out great quantities of urine. Still, the quantity and quality of urine can supply you with clues.

In fact, quantity provides the best clues when weighed equally with quality, which includes specific gravity, pH, color, odor, turbidity, and the presence of glucose, hemoglobin, or protein.

A question of quantity

The normal volume of urine voided by an adult in 24 hours ranges from 750 to 2000 ml, the average volume being about 1500 ml. But you have to temper the case to the circumstance, of course. For example, if you are doing a 24-hour urine collection on a patient who is NPO in preparation for a radiologic study, you've got to expect his urine output to be lower than usual.

Polyuria, the increased excretion of urine, is the physiologic response to several things: increased fluid intake, diuretic medications, and certain diuretic drinks such as coffee, tea, or alcohol. It can be produced by cold and by stress as well. But polyuria also occurs in several disease states such as uncontrolled diabetes mellitus and diabetes insipidus. (In the former, urine is highly concentrated; in the latter, very dilute.) Or polyuria can be an early sign of chronic renal failure indicating a loss of concentrating ability by the kidneys.

Oliguria, decreased urinary output, can take the extreme form of anuria, a total lack of urine. Physiologic forms of oliguria occur with decreased fluid intake, increased ingestion of salt, and excessive sweating. Oliguria also results from excessive loss of body fluid as in vomiting, diarrhea, or draining wounds. But then it happens, too, as a symptom of renal shutdown in either acute or chronic renal failure. If oliguria is extreme and sudden, it most commonly means mechanical obstruction to urinary flow.

A quality product?

The specific gravity of urine indicates the relative proportion of dissolved solids in it. You can easily measure specific gravity on the clinical unit with a Urinometer (a hydrometer) and a cylinder. Under standardized conditions, when fluids are either restricted or forced, specific gravity measures the ability of the kidney either to concentrate urine or dilute it. Normal specific gravity is between 1.005 and 1.030.

A very dilute urine can be an early symptom of renal failure. It can mean that because of tubular disease (e.g., pyelonephritis), the kidneys can't concentrate the urine sufficiently well to remove the normal quantity of waste solutes. To test

COLOR VARIATIONS IN URINE	
COLOR	**CAUSE**
Straw colored (dilute urine)	Nervous conditions, diabetes insipidus, granular kidney, large fluid intake
Dark yellow or amber (concentrated urine)	Acute febrile diseases, small fluid intake, vomiting, diarrhea
Turbid or smoky	Blood, chyle, spermatozoa, prostatic fluid, fat droplets
Red or red-brown	Porphyrin, hemoglobin, myoglobin, erythrocytes, transfusion reaction, hemorrhage, bleeding in urogenital tract, pyrvinium pamoate (Povan)
Orange-red or orange-brown	Drugs such as phenozyopyridine (Pyridium), urobilin
Yellow-brown or green-brown	Jaundice, obstruction of bile duct, phenol poisoning
Dark brown or black	Methylene blue medication, chorea, typhus
Cloudy	Pus, blood, epithelial cells, fat, phosphate bacteria, colloidal particles, urates, all-vegetable diet

this the patient may be ordered to be deprived of all fluids for 16 hours or overnight; the specific gravity should rise to 1.025 or more. A dilution test, less easy for the patient, can follow from the concentration test. The patient must drink 1000 to 5000 cc of water in a very short time, say, half an hour, and then empty his bladder at intervals between 1 and 4 hours later. The specific gravity should normally fall to about 1.002, and all water be excreted.

A condition to be ruled out when the patient voids quantities of watery urine is diabetes insipidus. This disease, by affecting the pituitary, impairs or even prevents secretion of antidiuretic hormone, ADH. Though great amounts of water are drunk, they are wasted, and the urine has a specific gravity no higher than 1.001 to 1.003.

Specific gravity rises, and urine becomes concentrated, in patients with diabetes mellitus, adrenal insufficiency, hepatic disease, and congestive heart failure. It is high whenever there has been great loss of water through sweating, fever, vomiting, or diarrhea. A word of warning: The contrast media used in X-ray studies can produce an exceptionally high specific gravity (greater than 1.040). So if your patient's urinary specific gravity is that high, check first to see if he has had a study within the past day or two.

The pH of the urine measures its hydrogen ion concentration. A pH below 7 indicates acidic urine; a pH above 7, an alkaline urine. Normal kidneys can produce urine that varies from a pH of 4.5 (highly acidic) to slightly above 8.0. Normal, freshly voided urine from patients on normal diets is acid, with a pH of about 6.0. Excessively acidic urine, with a pH below 6.0, may come from a high-protein diet, acidosis, uncontrolled diabetes mellitus, or certain medications such as ammonium chloride and mandelic acid.

Alkaline urine is frequently excreted after meals as a normal response to the secretion of hydrochloric acid in the gastric juice. In other words, as the body temporarily gives up gastric acid into the digestive bolus, the kidneys excrete a corresponding amount of bicarbonate as a compensation. Diets high in vegetables, citrus fruits, and milk and other dairy products can produce alkaline urine. Certain medications, such as sodium bicarbonate, potassium citrate, and acetazolamide also can cause alkaline urine. Defects in hydrogen excretion in the kidney, such as renal tubular acidosis and Fanconi's syndrome, a condition where solutes enter the urine in excess because of impaired tubular absorption, result in a neutral urine pH that never falls below 6.0 even with systemic acidosis. You can easily measure urine pH with nitrazine paper and a color chart.

The color of the urine provides useful clues about the substance within. Color intensity can indicate urine concentration: A dark color may indicate a dense urine; a pale color, a dilute urine. Comparing this with the fluid intake can give you information on the kidney's concentrating abilities.

Urine's color can change in the presence of pigments that occur in some disease states. Bile pigments, an early sign of liver disease, can produce a yellow to yellow-brown or greenish color. The porphyrins produce a dark brown-red color upon standing; hemoglobin gives a reddish-brown one. The urine will take different colors following ingestion of various dyes, foods, and drugs.

Freshly voided urine has a characteristic odor. After urine has stood for any length of time, it normally develops an ammoniacal odor from the decomposition of urea. But you may notice other odors. If a diabetic patient is spilling ketones, for example, the urine will take on a fruity odor; this is acetone. In patients with urinary tract infections, the urine may smell foul, especially when the infecting organism is a

Sweaty feet or acidemia?
You can tell much about a patient's renal function just from the odor of his urine. Here are some characteristic odors and their causes:
Mustiness — phenylketone
Sweaty feet — isovaleric, butyric, or hexanoic acidemia
Stale fish — trimethylamine
Vinegar or yeasty dough — decomposition of diabetic urine
Rotten egg — cystine
Feces — fecal contamination of the urine

coliform bacillus. With urinary tract infections, also, abnormal turbidity may be found; this is usually owing to its alkalinity rather than to the actual number of bacteria or leukocytes it contains.

A detectable amount of glucose in the urine — glucosuria — occurs whenever the blood glucose level exceeds the reabsorption capacity of the renal tubules. Glucosuria can sometimes be benign; you would expect it after a heavy meal or emotional stress. But the most common cause is diabetes mellitus. You can easily measure glucose in the urine on the clinical unit with a Clinitest reagent tablet or a reagent strip such as Tes-Tape (see NURSING SKILLBOOK *Managing Diabetics Properly*).

When hemolysis occurs somewhere in the body, free hemoglobin is released. If hemolysis occurs in the bloodstream, as with hemolytic anemia, free hemoglobin enters the blood. With a sufficient quantity of it, significant amounts enter the glomerular filtrate and appear in the urine. Red blood cells can also enter the urine at any point in the urinary tract as a result of disease or trauma. When this happens, they hemolyze in the urine itself, releasing detectable amounts of free hemoglobin. Again, you can easily detect the presence of hemoglobin with a reagent strip such as Hemostix.

Frothy urine may indicate abnormal protein excretion. Normally between 40 and 80 mg of protein are excreted in the urine each day, although as much as 100-150 mg per day may be within normal limits. This wide range in the so-called normal values comes from biological variations as well as differences in methods used for determining protein. But any amount higher than 150 mg indicates certain proteinuria. And that is an important indicator of renal disease. Two factors determine the amount of proteinuria: the precise nature of the clinical and pathological disorder causing it, and the severity of that specific disease. Severe proteinuria is often accompanied by edema. You can measure protein in the urine simply by using a colorimetric reagent strip such as Albustix.

As you can see, you can readily assess many facets of renal function. Dysfunction in the renal system can bring serious consequences to the patient. But if you are alert, you can often detect problems early enough to correct them. Sometimes you can prevent the problems entirely.

SKILLCHECK 4

1. Ralph Reeder, a 57-year-old construction worker, has been brought to the E.R. with sudden onset of severe pain in his back and right side. He is diaphoretic and complaining of nausea. His vital signs are: B.P., 130/90; pulse, 100; respiration, 28. After his examination, the doctor diagnoses renal calculi.

What findings would you expect in a nursing assessment?

2. Bob Blackmore has been admitted to the CCU after abdominal surgery. On his second day post-op, you notice that his urinary output has fallen to 500 cc over the past 24 hours; in the last 2 hours, he has been anuric.

What nursing assessments would you make?

3. Pam Galt, a 22-year-old diabetic, calls the office complaining of burning when she urinates. What questions would you ask Pam?

4. Vincent Douglas has been brought to the E.R. after an automobile accident in which he hit another car from the rear. You find his vital signs to be: blood pressure, 90/60; pulse, elevated; respiration, shallow and regular, with crepitus over the left lateral rib.

Mr. Douglas complains of pain in the left upper quadrant. Based on X-rays, a physical exam, and lab work, the doctor diagnoses spleen rupture, left lateral rib fracture, and hypovolemia.

What would your assessment probably reveal?

5. Marlene Jacobs, a 60-year-old chronic alcoholic, has arrived at the emergency room complaining that her "belly is swollen and getting bigger." Based on a chest X-ray, lab work, physical exam, and patient history, the doctor diagnoses ascites and chronic cirrhosis.

What findings would you expect in a nursing assessment?

6. Joan Rodriguez is an obese, 48-year-old mother of five. She has come to the hospital complaining of episodes of sudden, sharp pain in her right upper abdomen and of vomiting, especially after eating fried or fatty foods. Blood work and X-rays confirm the doctor's diagnosis of acute cholecystitis.

What findings would you expect in a nursing assessment?

7. Daniella Brown, 16 years old, developed severe abdominal pain at school and was sent home. Shortly after arriving home, she began vomiting. The family doctor advised her mother to take Daniella to the emergency room. There, based on a patient history, physical exam, and lab work, the doctor diagnosed acute appendicitis.

What signs and symptoms would your nursing assessment most likely turn up?

(answers on page 184)

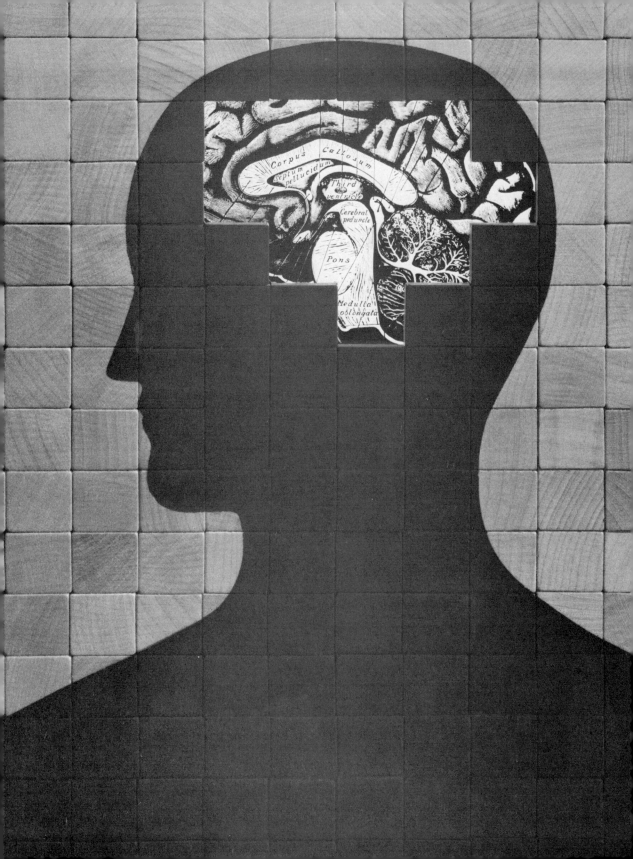

ASSESSING CRANIAL FUNCTION

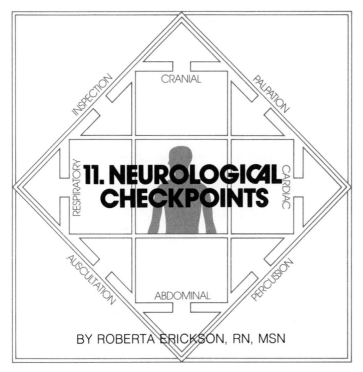

11. NEUROLOGICAL CHECKPOINTS

INSPECTION · CRANIAL · PALPATION · RESPIRATORY · CARDIAC · AUSCULTATION · ABDOMINAL · PERCUSSION

BY ROBERTA ERICKSON, RN, MSN

AN ACCIDENT VICTIM WITH severe head injuries...a teenager who has OD'd...a woman in a diabetic coma...a factory worker who has inhaled toxic fumes...an elderly man who has had a stroke — these are some of the patients whose nursing care will call for repeated neurological assessments.

In some of these cases, your skill in promptly recognizing and accurately interpreting changes in levels of consciousness and other neurological symptoms could mean the difference between your patient's developing irreversible brain damage or his recovery.

Here, then, is a review of checkpoints for a basic neurological assessment.

Loss of consciousness means brain failure just as uremia means renal failure. To be conscious, a person needs an intact brainstem reticular formation with nerve pathways to at least one side of his cerebral cortex. These brain areas can be impaired by increased intracranial pressure or by noncerebral diseases that have harmful secondary effects on brain metabolism.

Pressure. We have a "boxed-in" brain. The rigid cranial bones leave little room for expansion of the blood, cerebrospi-

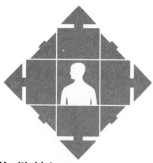

Health history:
What you should know
1. Does the patient have a history of neurological problems? Did he have surgery, injuries, or trauma? What treatments and medications did he use? Does he have allergies or hypertension?
2. Does he suffer from pain, fainting, dizziness, loss of memory, mood swings, seizures? Does he have trouble with hearing, vision, swallowing, fatigue?

nal fluid, and brain tissue inside. An increase in the volume of any one of these takes place at the expense of the other two, creating pressure that interferes with proper working of nerve cells and, ultimately, permanent loss of function. That's why early recognition is vital.

Some conditions that can lead to increased intracranial pressure are: a tumor, abscess, or cerebral edema (more brain volume); an epidural, subdural, or intracerebral hematoma (more blood volume); and hydrocephalus (more cerebrospinal fluid volume).

Metabolic causes of altered brain function accompany many kinds of illnesses and work in several ways. Hypoxia and hypoglycemia deprive the brain of oxygen and glucose respectively. Interference with blood flow (as in a stroke due to vascular occlusion) blocks the supply of both substances. Fluid, electrolyte, and acid-base imbalances alter nerve cell excitability. Internal toxins, in conditions such as liver or kidney failure, or external toxins, such as alcohol or depressant drugs, also induce brain malfunction.

Four groups of observations make up a practical assessment of brain function. They are: level of consciousness, ability to move, pupil responses, and respiration and other vital signs.

Level of consciousness
The single most important indicator of a patient's brain function is his level of consciousness (LOC). It ranges from alert wakefulness with full and appropriate response to stimuli to deep coma with no apparent responsiveness at all. Stupor, confusion, coma, and other terms used to label changes in consciousness can often be misinterpreted. Simple, accurate descriptions of the patient's behavior are much more useful.

Consciousness is perhaps most easily assessed in the order in which it deteriorates. That order is generally quite consistent, although no two patients will behave in exactly the same way. In the first four stages, your assessment will be primarily verbal — talking with the patient, asking him questions, having him carry out requests.

1. Is he alert and wakeful? A fully conscious person is aware of himself and his surroundings. You can get his attention easily or, if he's asleep, you can wake him without difficulty. He is well-oriented to his environment and responds appropriately to requests and events. Take sensory depriva-

tion into account, however, since even an awake, alert patient may lose track of the time of day or exact date during hospitalization. If the patient is not alert, continue the assessment.

2. Is he lethargic or restless? Early changes in consciousness can be subtle and might be overlooked unless you are alert for them and have a baseline for comparison. The patient may be only a bit more drowsy than usual or show less interest in what is going on. It's harder to get his attention or wake him up, and he takes longer to respond. On the other hand, the patient initially may be restless or irritable. Either lethargy or restlessness can progress to lower levels of consciousness.

3. Is he oriented? The four kinds of orientation are usually lost in a step-by-step order. The patient first becomes disoriented to time and cannot tell you the correct month and year. Second, he becomes disoriented to place and no longer knows where he is, or thinks he is someplace else. Daytime disorientation is more ominous since patients would first tend to have difficulty staying oriented at night. Third, he becomes disoriented to person and does not recognize family members and friends or may mistake them and you for someone else. Asking him to say your name may not be particularly helpful; better grounds for assessment would be asking the name of someone with whom he has had a long personal attachment. Fourth, he becomes disoriented to himself and does not respond to his own name and cannot tell you who he is.

Questions like "What is the month and year," "Where are you now," and "Tell me your name" may seem silly to a patient who *is* oriented. You may want to explain that you are going to ask him some simple questions to help you to know how he is.

4. Does he respond to simple commands? Ask the patient to do such things as squeeze your hand, raise his arm, wiggle his toes, blink his eyes, open his mouth, stick out his tongue, or touch his ear. Try him with several different commands — one at a time — and involve both sides of his body. If he has a hemiparesis or hemiplegia, paralysis rather than lowered consciousness may account for his inability to respond. If the patient is unresponsive to verbal stimuli, then go on to the next stage.

5. Does he respond to pain? Use just enough pain to be effective. One useful technique is to apply supraorbital pressure. Put your thumb under the notch in the bony orbit above

Categories of impaired consciousness

Defining every point on the spectrum between full consciousness and complete unconsciousness would be cumbersome — and futile. But the following classifications may serve as a useful guide.

FULL CONSCIOUSNESS (ALERT WAKEFULNESS)
Patient is fully aware of his surroundings, that is, oriented to time, place, and person; he responds appropriately to auditory, visual, and somatosensory stimuli.

DROWSINESS
Lethargy: Patient is inactive, indifferent; he responds slowly or incompletely to stimuli. Although capable of verbal responses, he may ignore some stimuli entirely. *Obtundation:* Patient is very drowsy and very indifferent; although capable of remaining awake, he may appear to be asleep.
Confusion and *delirium* describe consciousness impaired to about the same degree of drowsiness, but they imply thinking and behavior aberrations due to cortex dysfunction. The confused patient is disoriented and appears dazed; the delirious patient is uncooperative and easily agitated.

STUPOR
Patient can be aroused only by a continuous painful stimulus.

COMA
Response to intense stimuli is rudimentary or reflex (moderately deep coma) or absent (deep coma).

the patient's eye (about a third of the way from the inner corner) and press upward firmly. Other techniques: Apply pressure to the sides of his fingertip, put pressure on his fingernail by laying a pen or pencil across the nail, firmly pinch the trapezius muscle ridge between his neck and shoulder, or pinch the inside of his thigh or upper arm (best just above his elbow). Try these on yourself to appreciate the stimulus you're giving the patient. You may prefer not to roll your knuckles back and forth on the patient's sternum since bruising occurs easily there.

Again, the level of response descends in steps. At first the patient responds purposefully, by trying to withdraw from the stimulus or push it away from him. Next he responds nonpurposefully; he may only grimace or move his arm or leg in an irrelevant fashion. Finally, he fails to respond, as he slips into a very deep coma. Record the kind of stimulus you used and how the patient reacted, for example, "Grimaces and flexes right toes in response to supraorbital pressure."

6. Does he have corneal and gag reflexes? Reflexes are among the last responses to go, so for the patient's safety, specifically check for two of the cranial nerve reflexes. Occasionally test for the corneal reflex by holding each eyelid open in turn and lightly stroking his cornea with a wisp of cotton. He should blink immediately. Frequent checking is inadvisable, as this can irritate his cornea. Absence of corneal reflex calls for eye care to prevent drying and irritation.

The gag reflex is tested by holding down his tongue with a wooden depressor and touching the back of his pharynx on each side with the end of the depressor or a small cotton swab. Even with a gag reflex, however, the patient may be unable to handle his own secretions, so proper positioning and suctioning are needed to prevent aspiration and airway obstruction.

Ability to move
Injury to almost any part of the nervous system affects a person's ability to move in some way. Therefore, changes in motor function give important clues to help determine the area of damage.

Observe whether the patient can move all four extremities. If you haven't already seen him do so spontaneously, ask him to move them. Check his grasp for strength, equality, and ability to release. Bring out subtle arm weakness by testing for

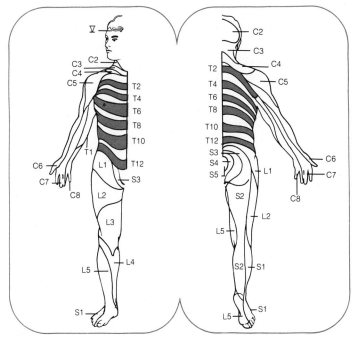

The paths of pain

When dorsal nerve roots are irritated, they produce pain all along the anatomical distribution of the affected roots. The area of skin supplied by a dorsal nerve root is called a dermatone. Using dermatones, as shown at left, you can trace abnormal skin sensations back to the spinal cord segment that causes the disorder.

pronator drift. Have the patient hold his arms in front of him with the palms up and ask him to close his eyes. A weak arm will drift slowly downward with his hand turning prone into a palm-down position. If the patient does not respond to these simple commands, then see if a painful stimulus will cause movement. Be sure to apply stimuli to both sides of his body. This will help you to rule out sensory impairment and to make comparisons.

If he doesn't respond to pain, you can still check for motor function. Raise his arms and let them fall back to the bed; the paralyzed arm will fall faster than one that is unaffected. To test his legs, flex them with his heels on the bed. When released, the paralyzed leg falls to the outside while the unaffected leg stays in place momentarily and then goes back to its original position.

Check the movement of facial muscles. Ask the patient to smile, show you his teeth, wrinkle his forehead, shut his eyes tightly, and open them. If necessary, apply supraorbital pressure. Watch for weakness or asymmetry: drooping of one corner of the mouth, drooling, uneven wrinkling of forehead, drooping of eyelid (ptosis), or inability to close eyelid tightly.

Watch for any unusual movements, and clearly describe them. For example, decorticate or decerebrate rigidity may occur spontaneously or in response to pain. In decorticate movement, which accompanies damage above the brainstem to the corticospinal (pyramidal) motor tract, the patient's legs are stiffly extended and his arms sharply flexed on his chest. In decerebrate posturing that occurs with upper brainstem damage, all his extremities are rigidly extended and his arms hyperpronated. Sometimes fragments or combinations of these responses occur.

Watch for unusual movements similar to the behavior of a young infant, such as reflex sucking or grasping. Avoid mistaking these for voluntary responses; they must be reported. Yawning, vomiting, or hiccoughing can occur with damage to certain lower brainstem areas. Some patients may have flaccid extremities without movement; others may have seizure activity. Both abnormalities need to be described carefully.

This is a good place in the cranial check to test for a Babinski sign. Stroke upward along the outside of the sole of each foot with a moderately sharp object like a key or pen top. The normal response is a downward bending (plantar flexion) of the big toe. When the big toe bends upward (dorsiflexes) instead, the Babinski sign is present. This is a normal reflex up to about 18 months of age, but is abnormal after that time, and indicates pyramidal tract malfunction. It is not necessary to stroke completely across the ball of the foot, which may be sensitive and cause a confusing withdrawal movement. Explain to the patient that you are going to rub the bottom of his foot and ask him to try to keep his foot still while you do.

Eye responses

The brainstem areas that help control consciousness are anatomically close to those that regulate pupil responses. Therefore, changes in the pupils and eye movements may suggest brainstem damage.

Keep in mind that nurses disagree about the importance of pupillary changes and, in fact, as to whether any change took place in a patient. Errors nearly always come from exaggerating the importance of changes. Nonetheless, you should always notify a doctor if you are sure that pupillary dilation exists, since emergency treatment may be needed.

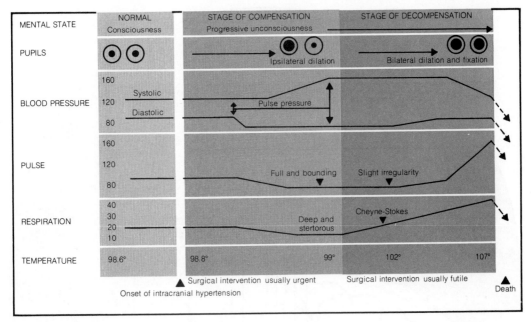

MENTAL STATE	NORMAL Consciousness	STAGE OF COMPENSATION Progressive unconsciousness	STAGE OF DECOMPENSATION
PUPILS		Ipsilateral dilation	Bilateral dilation and fixation
BLOOD PRESSURE	160 Systolic 120 Diastolic 80	Pulse pressure	
PULSE	160 120 80	Full and bounding	Slight irregularity
RESPIRATION	40 30 20 10	Deep and stertorous	Cheyne-Stokes
TEMPERATURE	98.6°	98.8° 99°	102° 107°

Surgical intervention usually urgent   Surgical intervention usually futile

Onset of intracranial hypertension   Death

First, observe the appearance of the patient's eyes by holding both his eyelids open and inspecting his pupils for their shape, size, and equality. Normal pupils are round and usually at a midpoint diameter within their range of about 1 to 9 millimeters. Although pupil size is commonly described using terms such as pinpoint, constricted, midpoint, or dilated, actually measuring the diameters with a small pocket ruler marked in millimeters will make the observation more specific. Remember that the size of normal pupils varies a great deal and that some people normally have unequal pupils. To interpret your observations, it helps to know what is normal for your patient — for example, by recording baseline measurements in the nursing history.

Next, assess the reaction of the pupil to light, preferably in a somewhat darkened room, using a small bright flashlight. To elicit the direct light reflex, hold each of the patient's eyelids open in turn and shine the light directly into his eye. This should cause a brisk constriction of his pupil. If the reaction is sluggish or his pupil remains fixed, the response is abnormal. Also test for the consensual light reflex. Hold both eyelids open, shine the light into one eye, and watch his other one. His

The perils of pressure
The above chart shows the changes in mental state, pupil dilation, and vital signs that accompany a fatal increase of intracranial pressure.

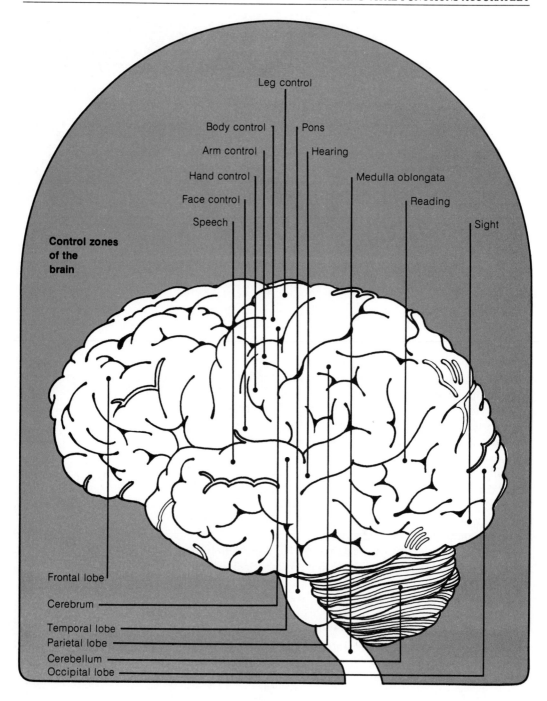

Control zones of the brain

Leg control

Body control

Arm control

Hand control

Face control

Speech

Pons

Hearing

Medulla oblongata

Reading

Sight

Frontal lobe

Cerebrum

Temporal lobe

Parietal lobe

Cerebellum

Occipital lobe

opposite pupil should also constrict, indicating intact nerve connections between the brainstem areas that regulate the pupils' constriction. An abbreviation sometimes used to record part of the pupillary finding is PERLA — pupils equal and reactive to light and accommodation.

Several situations interfere with assessment for pupil changes related to intracranial pathology. For example, don't be misled when direct injury to the eye affects the appearance or function of the patient's pupil. There is little value in checking his pupil if his eye is severely swollen. And, of course, if he is blind, his affected eye(s) will not react to light since the sensory part of the reflex pathway is absent. A slow or minimal pupil response to light can be hard to detect. If you're unsure of what you see, don't hesitate to have another nurse double-check.

Next, note any unusual eye movements. The eyes of an awake, alert patient are in parallel alignment, look straight ahead at rest, and make no involuntary movements. The same is generally the case in unconscious patients, although their eyes often rove spontaneously in a slow, random fashion. Some observers misinterpret this movement, thinking the patient is "following me with his eyes." The patient's eyes should gaze and move together in a parallel fashion. Deviations occur when the extraocular muscles cannot function properly. Check extraocular movements by asking the patient to hold his head still and follow your finger with his eyes to one side, up and down, and then repeat on the other side. Abnormal eye movements include deviation of one or both eyes from midline, nonparallel (dysconjugate) gaze or movement, cross-eyes (strabismus) from bilateral deviation toward the center, and a back-and-forth oscillation (nystagmus).

Respiration and other vital signs

Of the four traditional vital signs, respiration is the most useful in assessing cranial function. The act of breathing is influenced by many different parts of the brain, and conditions that impair consciousness may cause respiratory changes as well.

Obviously, maintaining a clear airway rates the highest priority in caring for any patient, whether conscious or not. So make sure he *can* breathe before you begin any other observations. Keep the patient on his side with his head slightly downward to promote drainage of secretions and prevent his

Control zones of the brain
The figure on the opposite page shows the different zones of the brain and the functions each controls. An injury on the top of the head may not necessarily affect the functions of the cerebrum. Since the skull is unyielding, pressure shifts the brain tissue downward toward and ultimately through the tentorial notch. As the brainstem is compressed, the patient may suffer disturbances in leg or body control as well as sight.

tongue from falling back over the airway.

Describe the patient's breathing. Has the rate increased or decreased? Is the depth of respiration deep or shallow? Is the rhythm regular, irregular in some consistent pattern, or irregular with no observable pattern? One common consistent pattern is Cheyne-Stokes respiration, regular fluctuations between apnea and hyperpnea. But rather than trying to name the respiratory pattern, record a specific description. Rate alone is an inadequate assessment (see Chapter 1).

Changes in the patient's blood pressure and pulse are important, but the classic symptoms of a rising blood pressure and a slow pulse associated with increased intracranial pressure occur late and after consciousness already has begun to deteriorate. These changes are distinct from the clinical picture of shock in which the blood pressure falls while the pulse quickens. A person cannot lose enough blood into his cranial cavity to cause shock. Therefore, if you observe shock symptoms, look elsewhere in his body for the cause. (See Chapter 14.) One exception: A small infant *can* develop shock due to intracranial bleeding since his total blood volume is small relative to his cranial capacity.

Impaired brain function seldom causes significant changes in body temperature unless there has been direct damage to the temperature regulating center in the hypothalamus. A gradual elevation is likely to be an early sign of infection in the lungs, urinary tract, or a wound. Each rise in degree of temperature increases the brain's metabolic rate, adding further insult.

Communicating the findings
Some observations call for urgent medical attention. Here are some examples of changes that must be quickly reported to a physician:

• A patient suddenly begins to show symptoms of decreasing consciousness when none had existed before. Early recognition and treatment provide the best chance of halting deterioration before irreversible damage develops.

• A patient's deficits were previously limited to either a decrease in consciousness only, with no paralysis, or localized paralysis only, without a lowering of consciousness. Now he develops a decreased level of consciousness plus decorticate or decerebrate movements. This group of symptoms suggests

**CRANIAL CHECKS FOR 4-MONTH-OLD INFANT
WITH RIGHT SUBDURAL HEMATOMA**

8 a.m.:
No response to verbalization or loud noise. Does not cry or make other sound. Remains in continuous decorticate rigidity with back arched — rigidity increases in response to pain. No Babinski reflexes. No sucking, rooting, or grasp reflexes. Pupils equal at about 2 mm. Direct reaction to light brisk on R, sluggish on L. No consensual reaction to light. Respirations deep and regular at 28/minute with O_2 at 6 L/minute via trach collar. BP=146/78, P=120, T=98⁴.

12 noon:
Cranial check — same as above except both pupils show brisk direct reaction to light; consensual reaction present on L, none on R.

an expanding intracranial lesion causing enough pressure to impair nerve pathways between the cerebral hemisphere and the brainstem.

• A patient suddenly develops a fixed, dilated pupil. This also can mean an expanding intracranial lesion is producing enough pressure to push cerebral tissue through the opening in the tentorial membrane and compress brainstem structures below.

Remember: The level of consciousness will change before pupil responses or vital signs are affected, so make every effort to detect early signs before later, more ominous ones develop.

When communicating your observations, be sure to include the time and sequence of events, what symptoms occurred together, and what changes have taken place since the last check.

Some hospitals have developed special forms, or flow sheets, that facilitate consistent, concise recording. An example of narrative descriptions is shown on this page. On these forms you describe the entire set of cranial check observations at the initial assessment, and at least once each day at a relatively consistent time in any event. The Glasgow Observation Chart offers a slightly different approach. Using it, various staff members can be consistent in recording such data as eye opening, best motor response, and verbal response on a bedside graph. When a cranial check duplicates or approximates the preceding one, simply record that the check was done and the results were unchanged except for items noted.

One good time to do a cranial check is on nursing rounds at the change of shifts. Go to the patient's bedside with the oncoming nurse. Show him or her what stimuli you have used and share your descriptions of the patient's responses. Such sharing helps to keep cranial checks comparable around the clock.

How long does it take to do a cranial check? Once you have practiced carefully several times, you need only a few minutes. Try to make your observations in the same order each time. A consistent approach will help you make complete observations and become skillful more quickly.

Make a complete cranial check each time, if at all possible. If other priorities permit only a shortened version, include the most essential observations for the patient concerned. For example, if you are working with another patient in the room and need to know if your cranial-check patient is still alert and able to verbalize, call to him to ask how he's doing. If he answers quickly, appropriately, and shows awareness of his surroundings, you have a reasonable check of his level of consciousness.

How often should a cranial check be done? Make the first check as soon as the patient arrives, to establish a baseline for later comparison. For the patient with an acute head injury, stroke, or craniotomy, you may want to check as often as every 15 or 30 minutes. As the patient's condition becomes stable, you may extend the interval to 2, 4, or 8 hours. If significant changes occur, once again make checks more frequently — whether they are ordered or not. Continue the same schedule during the night. It is no kindness to the patient to let him sleep while he slips into unconsciousness. Continue the checks as long as changes are likely to occur. In the patient with a subdural hematoma, for example, symptoms can occur early or not for days or weeks.

The cranial check is an important addition to your tools for patient assessment. Make each check as if your patient's life and health depended on it. They very well may.

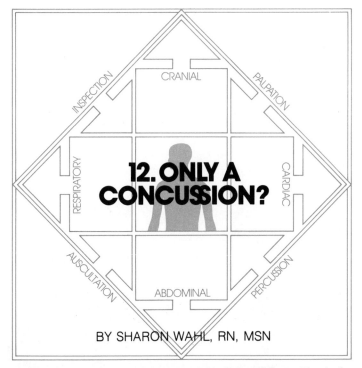

12. ONLY A CONCUSSION?

BY SHARON WAHL, RN, MSN

EVEN THOUGH CONCUSSION IS the mildest form of brain injury and the patient usually recovers spontaneously, you must be able to identify its symptoms. Because if you misinterpret the bizarre behavior that concussion often produces, you're likely to restrain and struggle with the patient. And straining or excitement will increase his blood pressure, which will increase intracranial pressure and risk further damage. The sad result: The patient, who had only a simple concussion, ends up in cerebral edema and serious sequelae as described in the preceding chapter.

To accurately assess a patient for concussion, you should understand the mechanics of head injury.

Head injury can be loosely categorized into two types: direct (a blow on the head) and acceleration-deceleration (indirect — as in an automobile accident when the victim's head snaps forward and then backward, jarring the brain).

In direct head injury, the skull protects delicate underlying brain tissue, absorbing much of the impact. Even so, shock waves are transmitted to the underlying moveable tissues. The degree of damage — from no injury or simple concussion to severe brain damage — depends upon several factors: the

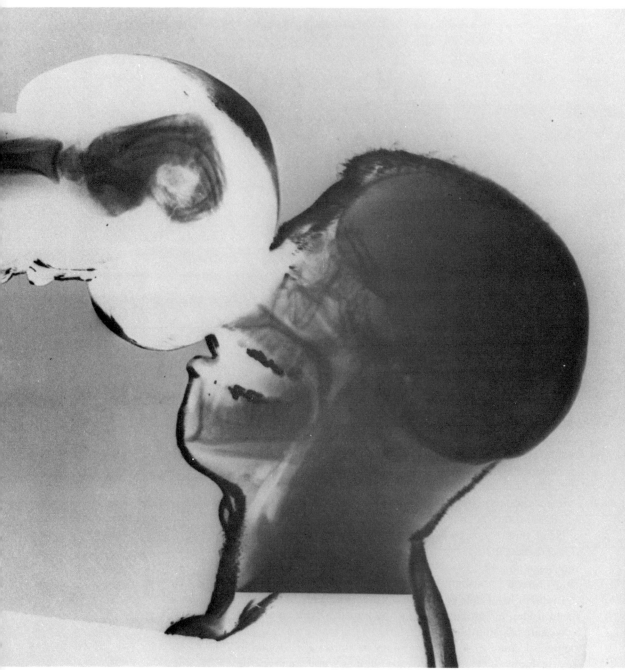

Howard Sochurek

force of impact, the type or quality of impact, and the location of impact. For example, locations susceptible to severe injury are the temporal area (which has a thinner bony covering and the middle meningeal artery close to the surface) and the base of the brain (where articulation with the cervical spine occurs).

Acceleration-deceleration head injury is more frequently seen in hospitals and in many cases is more serious. Inside the skull, the soft, watery brain contents jar against the bony ridges, the frontal and temporal-parietal being the most prominent. The brain subsequently rebounds against the opposite side of the skull — the coup-contracoup phenomenon. (Technically, this term is used in relationship to direct-blow injury. But the sequence of events occurring within the skull is comparable in acceleration-deceleration trauma.) Simultaneously, since the brain is on a short leash of tendons, nerve tracts, and blood vessels, shearing stresses occur. These shearing stresses cause the nerve fibers, vessels, and tendons in the brain stem to stretch, even rupture. The consequence of this mechanical and vascular trauma can be tissue shock, contusions or lacerations with hemorrhage, increased production of cerebrospinal fluid, and cerebral edema. Anyone who comes away from such an accident with only concussion is indeed fortunate.

What to look for

Like intracranial pressure, concussion may disturb the patient's level of consciousness; he may be dazed or, more commonly, become unconscious for a short time. But unfortunately for your assessment, concussion doesn't produce the other hallmarks of cranial injury: marked change in pulse, temperature, and respiration; muscle weakness or paralysis; and pupillary change. In fact, in nearly all cases the patient's vital signs remain completely normal.

So how do you identify concussion, particularly if the patient is only slightly dazed? You look for *behavioral* symptoms — those related to disruption of brain tissue in the frontal and temporal-parietal ridges. Disruption in the frontal lobe produces bizarre, irrational behavior. Some patients' behavior becomes immature and lacking in normal social restraint (i.e., swearing, combativeness, restlessness). Disruption in the temporal lobe produces temporary amnesia and disorientation. Thus, the patient may be unable to remember the acci-

Heads up
In head injuries the impact of the brain against the skull leads to concussion or contusion. The illustration on the opposite page shows what happens when a punch lands on a boxer's head. You can see how the brain has been momentarily forced to the back of the skull.

dent and will be disoriented to time and location.

Because of altered perception and memory loss, he may become frightened and confused when he finds himself in the strange environment of the hospital; he can easily misinterpret the actions of those trying to help him. You know how over-whelming an intensive care unit can be to an alert and aware patient. Imagine the terror it can engender in the disoriented patient. Little wonder that he reacts at a survival level — fighting back, crying for help. His loss of learned social control produces activity comparable in some ways to that of a 4-year-old child. The problem is that, unless you're alert to the possibility of concussion, you're apt to mistake these be-havioral changes for personality or emotional disturbances. The following case is typical.

A patient with a concussion

Mark Smith, age 17, was admitted to ICU from the emergency room at 6 a.m. with a head injury and possible concussion following an automobile accident. According to police, he was awake immediately after the accident, but lost consciousness shortly thereafter. On admission to the emergency room, the doctor noted that his neurological signs were within normal limits. Skull X-rays demonstrated no fractures or midline shift. Findings from blood studies including arterial gases were within normal limits.

When Joan Martin came on duty at 8 a.m., she noted his condition: blood pressure 120/80, pulse 100 and regular, respi-rations 24 and regular, pupils equal and reactive, movement capability in all extremities. He was responsive to verbal stimuli, but was drowsy.

By 8:30 a.m., he had changed dramatically; he had become very restless and was thrashing about in bed. Every few min-utes, he would sit up in bed, stare straight ahead and say, "Where am I? What happened?" Then he would lie down, appearing to sleep for short periods. Joan Martin told him where he was and why several times, but he stared blankly at her each time. At one point he cried, "I want my Mommy!" When she asked him to grip her fingers and reached for his hands, he suddenly struck out at her and directed a stream of profanity at her.

When she tried to grasp his wrists, he struck out again and

SIGNS AND SYMPTOMS IN HEAD INJURIES

CONCUSSION
Injury is functional
  mild   • transient loss of consciousness
          • possible impairment of higher mental
          functions, such as retrograde amnesia and
          emotional lability

  severe • prolonged unconsciousness
          • impairment of functions of brain stem,
          such as transient loss of respiratory
          reflex, vasomotor activity, and dilation of pupils

CONTUSION (bruising of the brain) and LACERATION (tearing of
  neural tissue)
  Injury is organic
          • prolonged loss of consciousness
          • lingering neurological deficit
          • frequent involvement of frontal and temporal
          cortices and midbrain
          • shock, headache, and vertigo in varying
          degrees
          • convulsions and focal damage such as
          monoplegia or hemiplegia possible
          • blood in spinal fluid

hollered, "What are you trying to do to me — kill me?"

Shielding herself, Joan called to another nurse, "This kid must be on drugs or something. Get the orderlies to help us tie him down before he hurts someone." As several nurses and orderlies descended upon him with restraints, Mark cowered in the corner of his bed looking like a trapped animal. After much yelling, hitting, scratching, and general confusion, he was finally tied down firmly, though he continued to struggle against his imprisonment.

"I'll get even with you...you'll pay for this!" he shouted after the retreating staff.

When Mark's parents arrived they were horrified at their son's behavior. They explained that, though Mark was a normally exuberant teenager, he was also an honor student and president of the high school student body.

Mark exhibited typical behavior for a person with a concussion. Unfortunately the staff reacted as most humans do when attacked verbally and physically, when they don't understand what is happening, and when they don't know how to handle the situation. Their failure to recognize the signs of concussion could have turned Mark's minor injury into a major one.

Once you've determined that a patient has suffered a concussion, you should frequently check his neurological status to make sure he doesn't slip into dangerous cerebral edema. Check vital signs, limb motion, and pupils as described in Chapter 11. Since the patient's anxiety or wild movements can interfere with an accurate assessment, you first must try to cope with the patient's combative behavior. In most cases, you can gain his cooperation if you first gain his trust by reorienting him each time with explanations of what you are doing. During your assessment, never make an unexpected or rapid movement toward the concussion patient. Don't touch him in a way that might be interpreted as restraining, such as holding his hands. And don't express value judgments about his behavior or reprimand him.

Of course, do not sedate any head-injury patient, especially with opiates, barbiturates, or diazepam (Valium). Sedation not only interferes with an accurate assessment of level of consciousness, but it also may cause respiratory depression resulting in carbon dioxide accumulation. Carbon dioxide, a powerful cerebral vasodilator, can increase cerebral edema and intracranial pressure.

By learning to recognize the behavioral signs and symptoms of concussion in a head-injury patient, you can respond with appropriate nursing care. That may well save him from a far more serious brain injury.

SKILLCHECK 5

1. Eight-year-old Mark Banner has been admitted for observation after a head injury. During your routine hourly check, you find him unresponsive and breathing quite noisily, with a noticeable expiratory grunt. His vital signs are: blood pressure, 130/60; pulse, 62; respiration, 25.

What do you think is happening to Mark?

2. Six hours ago, John Cannon was in an automobile accident in which he received possible head and internal injuries. During his first five hourly cranial checks, he had no unusual symptoms other than mild to moderate generalized pain. But this time you make these observations: Seems more drowsy and doesn't recognize where he is. Left arm and leg slightly weaker than right; no Babinski reflexes. Right pupil slightly larger than left. Direct and consensual light reflexes present bilaterally, though more sluggish on right. Blood pressure, 80/42; pulse, 110; respiration, 22 regular.

What do you think is happening to John?

3. Pattie O'Dell, 22 years old, was admitted today for observation after she fell while hiking and hit her head on some rocks. During the night shift, she has become increasingly upset at being awakened every hour for her cranial check. She cries, is uncooperative, and says she just wants to be left alone.

Would you wait longer between cranial checks so Pattie can get more sleep?

4. Susan, your neighbor's 4-year-old daughter, fell and hit her head while playing about 1½ weeks ago. She cried for a while at the time but otherwise seemed all right. Now her mother tells you that Susan has been having headaches and seems sleepy much of the time.

What advice would you give Susan's mother?

5. George Williams, a 33-year-old accountant, was admitted to the hospital after 3 weeks of flu-like symptoms: variable headache, nausea, and vomiting. About 2 weeks before admission, his neck had become stiff. When he arrived at the hospital, he complained of blurred vision, tingling of his toes and fingers, and severe headaches. He also said he was becoming very forgetful and was having trouble with minor computations at work.

Although Mr. Williams seemed somewhat apprehensive when he was admitted, he was alert. His only abnormal vital sign was a blood pressure of 170/102.

The doctor performed a Lumbar puncture and found bloody spinal fluid. He suspected a subarachnoid bleed of unknown etiology but couldn't confirm it with a cerebral angiography until Mr. Williams' blood pressure came down.

After five days of hospitalization, Mr. Williams' blood pressure was normal. A cerebral angiography revealed bilateral aneuryms of the posterior communicating arteries with vasospasm on the left side (probably at the bleeding site). The doctor scheduled him for surgery 2 days later, provided the vasospasms disappeared.

Today, the day of surgery, Mr. Williams was using the bedpan when he suddenly lost consciousness.

What assessments would you make?

(answers on page 185)

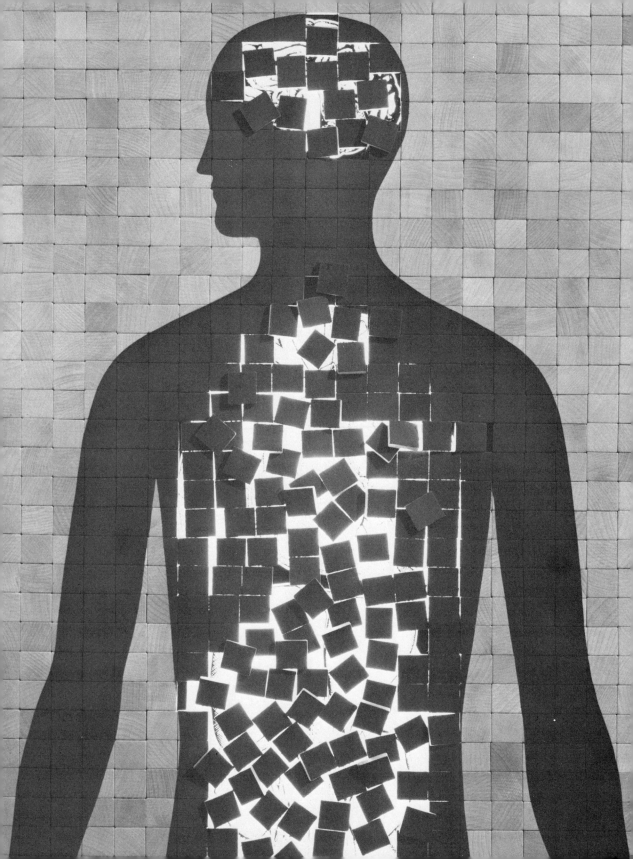

ASSESSING SHOCK

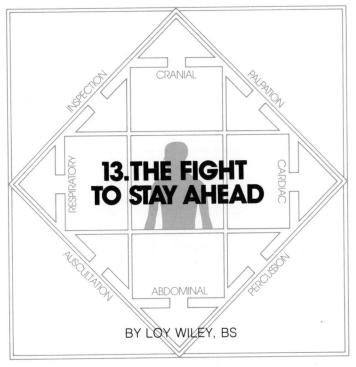

13. THE FIGHT TO STAY AHEAD

CRANIAL

INSPECTION

PALPATION

RESPIRATORY

CARDIAC

AUSCULTATION

PERCUSSION

ABDOMINAL

BY LOY WILEY, BS

THE FIRST FIVE SECTIONS of this book have dealt with the assessment of malfunctioning organ systems — one at a time. But your biggest assessment problem starts when all the systems malfunction at once. And the name of that problem is shock.

Hemorrhage, plasma loss from burned tissue, or dehydration from any cause eventually produces hypovolemic shock.

Dilation of veins and arterioles secondary to allergy or infection produces anaphylactic and septic shock.

Weak or inefficient heartbeat produces cardiogenic shock.

Whatever the initial event (and, thus, the classification of the shock), the compensatory responses that follow can affect the function of every organ system. Unfortunately, the body's compensatory system usually doesn't work: Septic shock kills 90% of its victims; cardiogenic shock, 80%. Hypovolemic shock kills a lower percent, chiefly because it develops more slowly and there's time to stay ahead. But with all three classes of shock, staying ahead is the only way you can beat the odds. How can you achieve the goal?

First, anticipate shock in any condition where it's likely: in trauma and burns and heart disease, in obstructed blood flow

Time after time
Staying ahead of shock means staying on top of changes in the patient's vital signs, intake, and output. And that means conscientiously measuring these functions every hour. Use a form such as the one shown here to keep track of your findings.

	DATE	12M	1am	2am	3am	4am	5am	6am	7am		8am
VITAL SIGNS	TEMP										
	PULSE										
	RESP										
	B.P.										
	C.V.P.										
	HEMATOCRIT										
INTAKE	ORAL										
	DEXTROSE										
	SALINE										
	HARTMANN'S										
	OTHER										
	BLOOD										
	PLASMA										
	HYPERIMMUNE SERUM										
	8 hrs TOTAL										
OUTPUT	URINE										
	EMESIS										
	OTHER STOOL										
	8 hrs TOTAL										
	SPECIFIC GRAVITY										
	SUGAR/ACETONE										
	PROTEIN/PH										
	NURSE'S NOTES										

or infection, in major endocrine, neuropathic, and metabolic disorders. Also watch for it in the very young, in the very old, and in the debilitated.

Second, stop thinking of the textbook case. You know: Mrs. Jones had cold, clammy skin; shallow breathing; rapid, thready pulse; reduced blood pressure; confusion; restlessness. That's shock, all right. But it's shock one step ahead of you. It's late shock.

Staying ahead of shock, then, means anticipation, accurate assessment, *early* recognition, and, of course, quick response.

Watch for change
Change, not absolute values, is the name of the game in assessing shock. Take blood pressure for example. The textbooks tell you a systolic blood pressure below 80 mm Hg indicates shock. In a hemorrhaging patient, it may also indi-

cate a 30 to 40% blood loss — and a 50% loss is usually fatal; in a hypertensive patient, it probably indicates advanced, irreversible shock. So, in a likely shock victim you need to watch for *patterns* of change: a slowly falling blood pressure, a slowly increasing pulse, rising carbon dioxide levels, decreasing urine output, increasing mental confusion, increasing irritability.

Where do you start when you see such a trend? Notify the doctor, of course, then start aggressive care. One way to remember your priorities in both assessment and treatment is to make your patient a VIP — very important, yes, but in this case the letters also stand for ventilation, infusion, and pump.

Ventilation rates priority in the patient in early shock because almost all shock patients develop tissue hypoxia. Oxygen-starved, these tissues must metabolize anaerobically, producing lactic acid as a by-product and, eventually, metabolic acidosis. Hyperventilation, an attempt to breathe off accumulating carbon dioxide, sometimes is the first sign of shock. It calls for immediate clearing of the airway; drawing of arterial blood for blood-gas measurements, CBC, type, and cross match; and starting oxygen by mask or airway to augment the oxygen-carrying capacity of arterial blood.

Why start oxygen right away? Don't the textbooks tell you to watch for cyanosis as the first sign of hypoxia? You can watch for it, sure, and it can be a lifesaver when it's the first sign. The problem is, the absence of cyanosis doesn't mean a thing. Some patients look pink and comfortable with a PaO_2 level of only 45 — a level at which arrhythmias become likely. Patients with preexisting heart disease are susceptible to arrythmias as soon as their PaO_2 falls below 80 — long before they appear cyanotic. So if you have other indications of developing shock, start oxygen. And remember that blood gas analysis, not skin color, is the only true measure of adequate tissue oxygenation. As we pointed out in Chapter 5, PaO_2 and $PaCO_2$ are the gases most frequently measured.

Still keeping an eye on ventilation — monitoring blood gases at frequent intervals to ensure that inhaled oxygen concentrations are keeping up with the body's demand — you should make infusion your next priority. Carefully monitor what goes in, what comes out, and how well it maintains circulating blood volume in between.

At the first hint of shock, start an I.V., insert a Foley, and

The tourniquet theory

No one fully understands the pathophysiology of shock. But one theory of septic and cardiogenic shock goes like this: Overdilation of the capillary beds creates a tourniquet-like effect, causing fluid to pool in the microcirculation and escape into the interstitial spaces. Without an adequate blood supply, tissues become anoxic and necrotic; gram-negative sepsis may further aggravate the condition to such an extent that the liver can't filter out the flood of toxins. Because of the large amount of bacteria in the bloodstream, the heart can develop bacterial endocarditis.

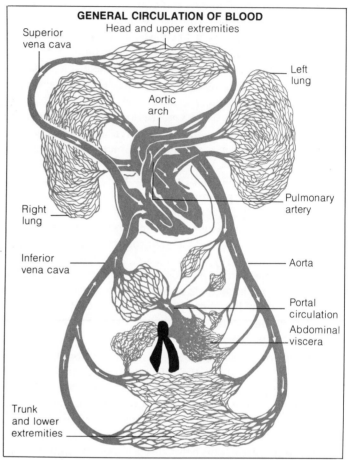

GENERAL CIRCULATION OF BLOOD

Head and upper extremities

Superior vena cava

Left lung

Aortic arch

Pulmonary artery

Right lung

Inferior vena cava

Aorta

Portal circulation

Abdominal viscera

Trunk and lower extremities

send a urine specimen to the lab for baseline levels.

The I.V. serves two main purposes: acute volume expansion to maintain adequate circulation while the patient is assessed and establishment of an intravenous line before peripheral veins shut down. Why give fluids when his blood pressure is fine? Unfortunately, in the shock patient peripheral blood pressure — like cyanosis — only tells you something when it's abnormal. In fact, a normal peripheral blood pressure may mean deepening shock! Let's see why.

Initially, blood pressure does indeed fall in all kinds of shock. In hypovolemic shock, pressure falls because of an absolute loss of fluid. In septic shock, it falls because of relative loss: Dilation of arteriole capacity (caused by circulating endotoxins) renders the circulating volume inadequate to fill the vascular system. And in cardiogenic shock, it falls because the pump is too weak to maintain adequate circulation, and blood pools in the venous system.

As capillary pressure falls, a kind of autotransfusion takes place: All along the capillaries, fluid is drawn in from the interstitial spaces, adding about a liter to circulating blood volume. (This flow into the capillaries also dehydrates the tissues, causing the thirst some patients develop in early shock.) If circulating blood volume is still inadequate, blood pressure continues to fall, and the body tries Plan 2: The sympathetic nervous system releases a barrage of chemicals to beef up the heart rate and constrict blood vessels in the skin, liver, lungs, intestine, and kidneys. The clinical signs of all this activity are clammy skin, oliguria, and a transient increase in blood pressure as circulation to the heart improves. Thus, a normal blood pressure accompanied by clammy skin and oliguria may indicate deepening shock. The patient obviously needs fluid replacement.

Measure ups and downs
To monitor the rate and quantity of the infusion, central pressure measurements are key since peripheral blood pressure is unreliable. Central venous pressure (CVP), pulmonary artery pressure (PAP) and pulmonary wedge pressure (PWP) can all be measured, but CVP is the easiest and most frequently used. (For a complete discussion of monitoring, refer back to Chapters 7 and 8.)

The problem with CVP monitoring is that the CVP may be normal despite hypovolemia if the body has compensated by constricting the peripheral vasculature. It also can be normal despite pulmonary edema secondary to fluid overload because the CVP doesn't accurately evaluate left-heart function.

Because of these limitations, many clinicians treat early shock aggressively with a fluid challenge: That is, they rapidly infuse a bolus of fluid, regardless of the initial CVP, and note the change in the CVP. If the rapid infusion improves blood pressure, urine output, and skin perfusion with little or no change in CVP, the patient needs fluids.

If the infusion causes a rapid elevation of CVP and no improvement, fluid overload is a danger.

During the fluid challenge, you must monitor the CVP con-

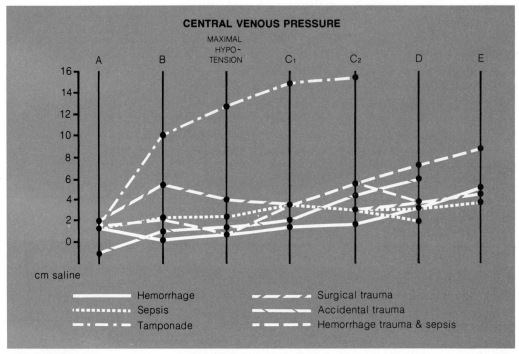

CVP patterns

CVP readings will vary widely from patient to patient, depending on the cause of shock. This chart shows the usual readings at various stages of shock. Stage A is the preoperative or pre-illness period; stage B, the initial period of falling arterial pressure; stages C_1 and C_2, the middle periods; stage D, the recovery period for surviving patients; and stage E, the pre-terminal period for terminal patients.

tinuously to prevent fluid overload, one of the most common complications of shock. As shock researcher Doctor Richard C. Lillehei once pointed out, fluid challenge is not "a license to drown the patient." Particularly if the CVP does not rise after replacement of 2 to 3 liters, you must determine that the CVP has not risen transiently, then dropped as fluid flowed into the lung or as continuing hemorrhage depleted the circulating volume again.

In some patients, the fluid needs of shock must be carefully balanced with the needs of other conditions. For example, following a suboccipital craniectomy for a cerebellar tumor, a 55-year-old patient's pulse was 110; systolic blood pressure, 100; and urine output 15 cc/hr. The recovery room nurse compared these with a preoperative pulse of 60 and blood pressure of 120, and called the neurosurgeon, who ordered 200 cc of ½NS/30 min. The pulse dropped to 90; blood pressure increased to 110; and urine output increased to 25 cc/hr.

Despite this response, which indicated hypovolemia, the neurosurgeon waited two hours before ordering another 200-cc bolus of fluids. Following this infusion, the pulse dropped to 70; blood pressure increased to 125; and urine output increased to 30 cc/hr. In this case, the neurosurgeon kept his patient on the thin edge of shock to minimize the possibility of brain swelling.

Patients with heart and lung disease also are particularly endangered by fluid overload, and in these patients the failure of the CVP to measure pressure in the left ventricle — the best representation of the heart's pumping efficiency — can be fatal. The PAP and PWP are far more reliable indicators.

Measure the ins and outs

What goes in must come out; and output is another valuable indication of the adequacy of fluid replacement. Output below 30 cc/hr indicates inadequate fluid replacement or a failing heart. Depending on other parameters, increased I.V. infusion and diuretics are indicated.

Unfortunately, quantity does not always indicate quality — in urine as in everything else. As we'll see in the next chapter, patients in septic shock and burn shock can actually urinate themselves to death. For this reason, repeated urinalyses are necessary. A trend toward increased creatinine and urea nitrogen values points to nonoliguric renal failure, and the doctor should be notified immediately. High urine sodium levels in a burn patient point to inadequate fluid replacement despite diuresis.

The third component of VIP is pump — a reminder that patients in shock from all etiologies must be assessed constantly for signs of pump failure. Pump failure is usually the cause of cardiogenic shock, but in septic and hypovolemic shock, it usually develops secondary to hypoxia. As we mentioned earlier, an arterial PaO_2 below 50 predisposes even a healthy heart to arrhythmias. Below 80, a diseased heart may develop arrhythmias. Obviously, it follows that close monitoring of the EKG for arrhythmias and repeated blood gas analyses — with prompt action if hypoxia seems to be developing — are key to preventing pump failure. Persistently low PaO_2 levels, despite oxygen therapy, indicate that oxygen transport across the alveoli is impaired, and assisted ventilation with a volume ventilator is required.

If your patient doesn't have a PAP or PWP line, watch the EKG, and palpate the femoral artery to assess cardiac output. A thready pulse indicates low pressure and signals the need for

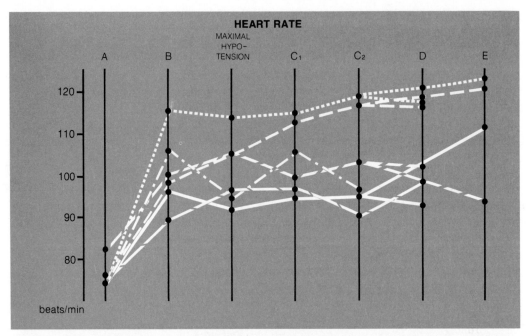

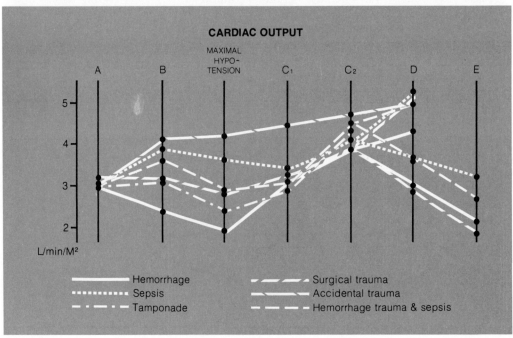

fluid replacement. A full pulse indicates adequate replacement or overload. Monitor the pulse for at least 30 seconds to determine irregularities in rhythm and rate. Distended jugular veins, dyspnea, cough, and rhonchi are other indications of pulmonary congestion and possible ventricular failure.

A varied course
Like CVP readings, cardiac output and heart rate generally follow patterns according to the type and stage of shock. The charts on the opposite page show you what to expect.

Medicate and monitor the effects

If all goes well, your assessment of ventilation, infusion, and pump efficiency — and your quick action when things start to go wrong — will prevent shock or reverse early shock. When all doesn't go well, a number of drugs may be used to reverse the effects of deepening shock.

Four major types of drugs are given in shock when supportive treatment fails: vasodilators to counteract the body's compensatory vasoconstriction; vasopressors to raise blood pressure either by stimulating heart rate and force or by peripheral vasoconstriction; diuretics to stimulate flow; steroids to combat adrenal insufficiency and inflammation.

As mortality figures indicate, no one drug regimen guarantees success, and the choice of drugs is often arbitrary. Here is a brief rundown on the drugs most often used in shock, their doses and effects.

Vasodilators may seem illogical in an already hypotensive patient, and their use has its dangers. The rationale is to counteract the vasoconstriction produced by the body's defenses. Obviously, aggressive fluid replacement must accompany administration of these drugs to satisfy the expanding circulatory system.

Phentolamine (Regitine), chlorpromazine (Thorazine), and phenoxybenzamine (Dibenzyline) are the peripheral vasodilators most often used in shock patients. During their administration, assess the patient frequently for adverse effects.

• Check the CVP. You may have to titrate the rate of flow of volume expanders to keep the CVP within the prescribed range.

• If CVP is not monitored, check blood pressure every 5 minutes. Stop the drug and increase fluids if systolic pressure drops below 70. Remember to keep the bed flat, since elevating the head may produce severe orthostatic hypotension.

• Assess and chart the patient's clinical condition and cardiac state frequently to indicate effectiveness of treatment.

Vasopressors are a mixed bag. Their desired effect is to

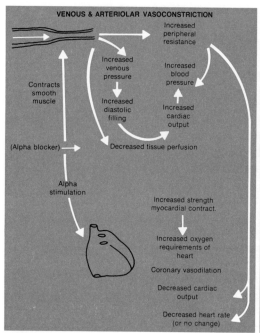

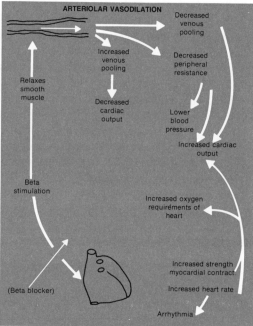

The alpha and the beta
In vasoconstriction, the venous and arterial smooth muscles contract, increasing peripheral resistance and blood pressure. This increases cardiac output.

In vasodilation, the smooth muscles of the arterioles relax, decreasing peripheral resistance and venous pooling. This, too, increases cardiac output.

increase blood pressure to increase circulating blood volume, but they may achieve this through heart stimulation alone, heart stimulation and peripheral vasoconstriction, or heart stimulation and peripheral vasodilation. The key to effective treatment is to increase perfusion — that is, to counteract the tissue hypoxia that accompanies shock. Thus, simple elevation of the peripheral blood pressure is ineffective if it is accomplished by constricting peripheral microcirculation alone.

Isoproterenol (Isuprel) and dopamine (Intropin) increase pressure by their direct effect on the heart while also dilating peripheral vessels. Both increase cardiac rate as well as force of contraction, and thus increase demands on the heart. Nursing assessments during administration of these drugs include:

• Monitoring EKG constantly. Isoproterenol can increase ventricular irritability. Keep defibrillator at bedside.

• Checking heart rate. Slow or stop infusion if heart rate exceeds 110/minute.

• Checking respiration.

• With isoproterenol, checking urine output and BP every 20 minutes.

Norepinephrine (Levophed), epinephrine (Adrenalin), and metaraminol (Aramine) have a vasoconstricting effect along with their direct cardiac effect. Nursing assessments with these drugs include:

• Monitoring EKG constantly. These drugs may cause arrhythmias in patients with heart rates above 120/minute.

• Watching for headache, chest pain or hypertension. Stop or slow drug and notify doctor if these develop.

• Checking for leakage. If it occurs, infiltrate tissue with phentolamine.

Glucagon and digitalis strengthen contractions without peripheral effects. Although they are chiefly used for patients in cardiac failure, some doctors use them in all forms of resistant shock. Nursing actions include:

• Monitoring pulse and EKG constantly. The digitalizing dose is extremely variable in shock patients, and toxicity risk is high.

• Watching for vomiting.

• Monitoring blood glucose frequently in diabetics.

Diuretics are sometimes administered early in shock to minimize the chance of acute tubular necrosis due to oliguria. Mannitol, furosemide (Lasix), and sodium ethacrynate (Edecrin, Lyovac) are the agents used most frequently.

• Monitor intake and output carefully.

• Monitor EKG and CVP constantly for early signs of hypovolemia.

• Once diuresis is established, monitor electrolytes frequently to maintain adequate potassium and sodium levels.

Steroids such as hydrocortisone, methylprednisolone (Solu-Medrol), and dexamethasone (Decadron, Hexadrol) are used widely in patients with septic shock, and, less often, in patients with cardiogenic shock. Although their value has not been proved conclusively, many doctors feel that their inotropic, vasodilating, and anti-inflammatory effects are beneficial, particularly if the steroids are given early in shock. Some clinicians give them for hypovolemic shock as well. Few side effects are likely after 1 or 2 bolus infusions of steroids.

With all the attention on the vital functions of a patient in shock, it's easy to forget the minor medical complications of shock. Yet relieving them is important in shock patients not only for compassionate reasons but also because shock patients have very little energy reserve. Here are some assessments to help you decrease demands on the patient's energy:

• Is the patient in pain? Pain exhausts the patient and can deepen shock. Relieve it promptly — but give reduced doses of sedatives and analgesics that depress respiration and remember that intramuscular injections do not provide predictable effects in patients with impaired circulation. Don't discount the effectiveness of reassurance and explanations to relieve apprehension and pain.

• Check for complications from stasis, such as respiratory difficulties and skin breakdown. If the patient is too brittle to be turned every 2 hours, tilt him from side to side, placing pillows under alternate sides. Encourage deep breathing, coughing, blow bottles, IPPB, and other measures that help maintain ventilation in all sections of the lung. For patients on volume respirators, frequent double breaths help keep lungs inflated. Exercise arms and legs and rub skin gently to reduce the risk of skin breakdown and increase circulation.

• Check the patient's skin temperature. Hypothermia increases hemoglobin saturation and thus decreases tissue oxygenation. Hyperthermia increases cell metabolism and demands for oxygen.

• Watch for other complications. There's very little that can't go wrong in shock. It's a truism that the shock patient is never stable: He's either getting worse or better. Assess all parameters frequently and carefully: Is there a change? Is the direction of change consistent? Is it accompanied by other changes? What could it mean? Watch, and act, and stay ahead.

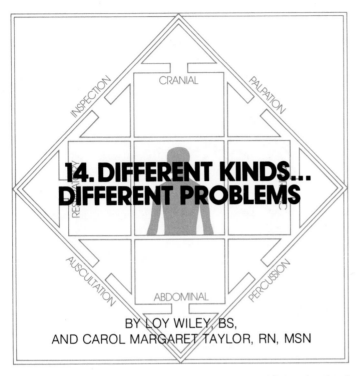

14. DIFFERENT KINDS... DIFFERENT PROBLEMS

BY LOY WILEY, BS,
AND CAROL MARGARET TAYLOR, RN, MSN

HYPOVOLEMIC SHOCK...SEPTIC SHOCK...cardiogenic shock
...each presents its own peculiar problems. The quicker you
recognize them — and act — the better the patient's chance of
survival. The critical nursing need is for assessment: to detect
the earliest sign of change in the quantity of circulating fluids
and the degree of tissue perfusion.

Loss of circulating fluid and reduction in tissue perfusion
are, of course, the underlying defects in all three kinds of
shock. The major difference is that hypovolemic shock is
initiated by a loss of circulating fluid. In the other kinds of
shock, the loss is secondary — to vasoconstriction in septic
shock, and to pump failure in cardiogenic shock.

Hypovolemic shock can be further classified according to
the condition causing the hypovolemia. The cause in adults
and school-age children is commonly either hemorrhage (due
to trauma or gastrointestinal disease) or thermal burns. In
contrast, the commonest cause in infants and small children is
diarrhea.

Patient history: Hemorrhagic shock
Bob G., a 24-year-old laborer, was admitted to the emergency

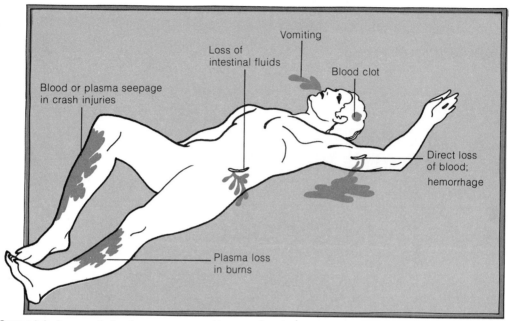

Loss of intestinal fluids

Vomiting

Blood clot

Blood or plasma seepage in crash injuries

Direct loss of blood; hemorrhage

Plasma loss in burns

Covert injuries, overt shock
Watch for hypovolemic shock in all trauma patients; they can lose fluids not only externally, through hemorrhage, vomiting, or burns, but also internally, through crush injuries or punctures of organs.

room at 7 a.m. after being struck by a car as he was walking across the street.

His only visible injuries were bruises on his left abdomen and chest and a deep laceration of one finger. During the examination, he sometimes became disoriented and restless. At times, he lapsed into semiconsciousness although his pupillary light reaction was normal and there was no history of head injury. His skin was pale and clammy; his pulse 144/min. His blood pressure was a normal 112/70 mm Hg.

How would you assess Bob G.'s condition and what would you do?

Realizing that the classic signs of shock seldom appear until shock is severe, many emergency departments assume every trauma victim is in shock until proven otherwise. They recommend the same initial treatment for all victims of trauma: resuscitation if the patient isn't breathing and his heart isn't beating; starting oxygen by mask or airway; starting an I.V. of D_5W or normal saline; moving the patient gently, keeping him horizontal to facilitate blood flow to the heart and brain; covering the patient with a light blanket; and inserting a Foley catheter. But they also recommend assessment for sure signs of shock:

• Recording the amount of blood lost.

- Recording urinary output.
- Inspecting the patient and recording vital signs every 15 minutes.

Except for massive arterial hemorrhage, hypovolemic shock generally deepens slowly, and several warning signs appear.

Skin changes reflect changes in tissue oxygenation and perfusion. Persistently cold, clammy skin during fluid replacement is a sign of continuing peripheral vascular constriction — an indication for faster fluid administration. If crystalloids are given slowly, they diffuse into interstitial space as fast as they are administered. Generally, all fluids are given rapidly until blood pressure rises to normal, then infusion is slowed to 40 drops per minute.

Flushing and sweating indicate overheating — a condition that increases the metabolic rate and the need for oxygen.

Persistent pallor and cyanosis in a shock patient generally indicate tissue hypoxia, but cyanosis in the lips and nail beds also occurs if the patient is cold. To avoid confusion, check for cyanosis (see Chapter 2) in an extremity that is lightly covered. Since change is key, the same person should evaluate cyanosis.

One note of caution: Good skin color is not proof of adequate tissue oxygenation. The only proof of tissue oxygenation is an arterial oxygen measurement.

Blood pressure and pulse require careful monitoring. Although blood pressure often stays normal until late shock, systolic blood pressure will eventually drop as much as 30 mm Hg as shock deepens. In hypertensive patients, the drop may not be apparent unless you know their usual blood pressure. One tip: If you suspect a patient is in shock despite normotensive readings, check for orthostatic hypotension. This develops before systemic hypotension in most patients with hypovolemia.

A drop in systolic pressure below 80 mm Hg generally indicates inadequate coronary artery blood flow, which may produce weak contractures and cardiac arrhythmias. When blood pressure drops this low, increase the oxygen rate and call the physician.

A progressive drop in blood pressure accompanied by a thready pulse generally indicates that fluid replacement is inadequate. A drop accompanied by a strong, rapid pulse or a strong, arrhythmic pulse generally indicates heart failure.

Depressing drugs
Although all narcotics can affect respiratory function, some are more dangerous than others. Morphine, hydromorphone (Dilaudid), and levorphanol (Levo-Dromoran) have the most potent effect, markedly depressing respiration. Codeine, however, has only about ¼ that effect on respiration and meperidine (Demerol) causes mild respiratory depression, bronchodilation, and sometimes bronchospasm.

Monitor the pulse for at least 30 seconds every 15 minutes to detect infrequent arrhythmias or changes in quality. If you can't detect a radial pulse because of peripheral vasoconstriction, use the femoral artery.

Occasionally, rapid pulse is the first sign of shock.

Respiration becomes rapid and shallow. Such air hunger is a common, early sign of shock as the body attempts to compensate for tissue anoxia. (Slow breathing — 2 to 3 breaths per minute — appears late in shock after failure of the compensatory mechanism.) Rapid, moist respirations during fluid replacement are a sign of pulmonary edema. When these develop, slow or stop the fluid infusion and call the physician.

Rapid, shallow breathing with cyanosis, despite oxygen administration, may be a sign of venoarterial shunting, called shock lung. This occurs when normally perfused secretions of the lungs are not fully ventilated, permitting unoxygenated blood to return to the left atrium.

Temperature usually drops below normal with hemorrhagic shock. Watch for change. A gradually increasing temperature should alert you to the possibility of developing sepsis. A gradual drop in temperature calls for another blanket or a warmer room temperature so that the patient doesn't exhaust himself trying to keep warm.

Restlessness is common in early shock and usually indicates hypoxia. If restlessness continues despite oxygen administration, fear and pain are likely explanations. Constant reassurances, explanations, and thoughtful gestures such as wiping the patient's face with a damp washcloth can go a long way toward relieving fear.

Relieving pain can be tricky since most narcotics depress respiratory function. If narcotics must be given, start with one-third the normal IM dose and give it slowly as an I.V. bolus, titrating the dose to the patient's response. If a patient was already receiving narcotics when he developed shock — for example, a postoperative patient — withhold all medications and call a physician.

Urine output below 30 ml/hr indicates a marked reduction in renal blood flow — a sign of severe shock. If uncorrected, ischemia may lead to renal failure. As soon as you notice a pattern of decreasing urine output, increase the fluid infusion rate to the maximum limit allowed and call a doctor.

Meanwhile back in the emergency room, what happened to

Bob? The staff instituted the steps we've just outlined. Laboratory reports showed a slightly depressed hemoglobin (13.8 Gm %). Specific gravity of the urine was 1.025, indicating mild concentration, probably secondary to internal bleeding. A CVP line was inserted, and pressure was maintained between 7 and 15 cm H_2O by varying infusion rates between 60 and 125 cc/hr.

Two hours after admission, the hemoglobin was down to 12.6, and Bob was agitated and incoherent. Urine output was 60 cc/hr; blood pressure was good; the pulse was 110 and thready. Bob's wife had announced that their religious beliefs forbade blood transfusions, and the staff continued to infuse a mixture of two-thirds Ringer's lactate and one-third low-molecular-weight Dextran with multivitamins and potassium chloride.

The patient was taken to the O.R. for a laparotomy, during which a ruptured spleen was removed. Vital signs remained strong postoperatively. The hemoglobin fell to 5.3 Gm % 2 days after surgery and still had not returned to normal at discharge, one month after injury.

As this case demonstrates, hemorrhagic shock can often be treated by fluid replacement alone if the bleeding is stopped, fluid replacement is prompt and adequate, and other complications do not develop.

In refractory shock, steroids, vasopressors, and other medications discussed in Chapter 13 are given.

Patient history: Burn shock
George R., 53 years old, was transferred from a community hospital 8 hours after he was burned. A cigarette had set fire to the couch on which he was sleeping, severely burning his right arm, chest, and abdomen. He was alert and in little pain. Blood was drawn for analysis, and a Foley catheter was inserted. An NG tube was inserted because burns of this size (greater than 20% of the body surface) are frequently associated with paralytic ileus. Ringer's lactate was started at 1 L/hr.

At the change of shift, the evening nurse noted that George seemed disoriented and restless. His vital signs and urine output were stable.

Restlessness is an important clue during the first 48 hours after a burn. With massive burns, skin color and temperature are often impossible to gauge. Furthermore, cold, clammy

Measure for measure

In gauging the severity of burns, you have to measure both the depth and size. When assessing depth, as shown on this page, remember:

• Erythematous areas that blanch with fingertip pressure and then refill are shallow partial-thickness burns (right portion of picture).

• Blisters (vesicles) usually indicate deeper partial-thickness burns (center portion), especially if they increase in size during the immediate postburn phase.

• Full-thickness burns (left portion) appear leathery, vary from white to brown or red or black, and produce no pain. They may produce small thin-walled vesicles but these won't increase in size.

To calculate the size of burns in adults, you can use the Rule of Nines shown on the opposite page. To estimate burn size in children, use the following table to adjust for differences in proportion:

Age	½ of the Head	½ of the Thigh	½ of the Leg
0	9½	2¾	2½
1	8½	3¼	2½
5	6½	4	2¾
10	5½	4¼	3
15	4½	4½	3¼

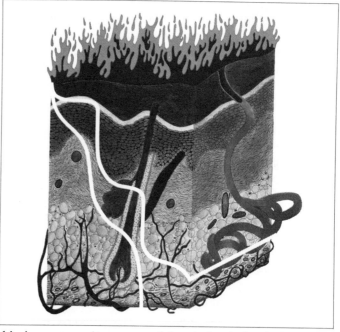

skin is common because peripheral circulation is frequently impaired by edema. Blood pressure and pulse often react *after* shock is established.

Sudden onset of mania and restlessness or disorientation during this period may be caused by discomfort, but it usually indicates hypoxia secondary to airway problems or shock because of inadequate fluid replacement. A sudden decrease in urine output also indicates inadequate fluid replacement and may presage shock. During the first 8 hours of resuscitation up to 10 liters of fluid may be required to restore an adequate blood volume and maintain an adequate urine output.

In George's case, the infusion rate was increased, and a CVP line placed to monitor circulating blood levels. Blood gases showed adequate oxygenation. Within 20 minutes his restlessness had disappeared. An alert assessment had prevented shock.

After the first 48 hours, neither mania nor urine output is a reliable sign of shock in burn patients. Patients frequently become disoriented and manic during this later period, perhaps to escape their pain and fear. And urine output may increase dramatically once diuresis begins. Cardiac output and

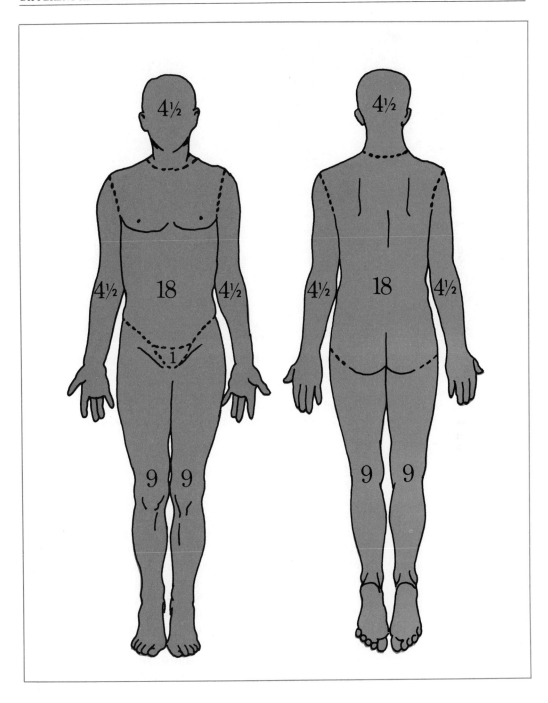

NORMS FOR VITAL SIGNS AND BLOOD GASES IN CHILDREN			
	0-1 YEAR	1-2 YEARS	2-3 YEARS	3-4 YEARS
BLOOD PRESSURE	90±25 systolic; 61±19 diastolic	96±27 systolic; 65±27 diastolic	95±24 systolic; 61±24 diastolic	99±23 systolic; 65±19 diastolic
PULSE	70-180	80-140	80-140	80-120
TEMPERATURE	99.6° F rectal; 98.6° F oral; 97.4° F axillary	99.6° F rectal; 98.6° F oral; 97.4° F axillary	99.6° F rectal; 98.6° F oral; 97.4° F axillary	99.6° F rectal; 98.6° F oral; 97.4° F axillary
RESPIRATIONS	30-40	28-32	28-32	24-28
BLOOD GASES	PaO_2 85-100 $PaCO_2$ 35-45	PaO_2 85-100 $PaCO_2$ 35-45	PaO_2 85-100 $PaCO_2$ 35-45	PaO_2 85-100 $PaCO_2$ 35-45

urine sodium levels become the most dependable gauges of adequate fluid replacement.

Special precautions: Infant diarrhea
In children 6 months to 3 years, diarrhea is the usual cause of hypovolemic shock. Treatment is often difficult because children can develop electrolyte imbalances so rapidly.

The signs of shock are essentially the same as for adults: cold, clammy skin; anxiety; and tachycardia. Hypotension, as in adults, may be a late sign.

Even more significant in small children and infants are sunken eyes and dry mucous membranes due to dehydration, which sometimes appear after only one day of diarrhea. In an infant, examine the testes or vulva. This skin will be wrinkled even when other signs of dehydration are absent.

There is an exception to this clinical picture, however. In hypertonic diarrhea, infants lose fluid but retain electrolytes — their serum sodium may climb to 160 mEq. (Normal for infants is 136 to 145 mEq/L.) The resulting edema may obscure the diagnosis unless you get a history of diarrhea and watch for other clues: doughy skin, elevated body temperature, central nervous system irritation and lethargy, seizures. These infants run a high risk of renal damage and cerebral bleeding if fluid replacement is delayed.

Once fluid replacement is under way, place a catheter, and draw blood for gases and electrolytes. Generally, a CVP line is put in, and EKG monitoring may also be necessary.

As with adults, constant assessment of vital signs is the key to caring for children in shock. Urine output should be greater than 10 cc/hr in the newborn to 3-year-old infant and 15 to 20 cc/hr in the 3- to 12-year-old child. The danger of renal shutdown secondary to high sodium levels is always present in hypertonic diarrhea.

Patient history: Septic shock

At 11 p.m., 62-year-old Anita R. was resting after a cystoscopic examination. The instrumentation was without incident, and the urologist found no infection or pathology.

Back from the recovery room about noon, Mrs. R. had complained of being chilled. Of course, this complaint often follows general anesthesia. Shortly afterwards, she had a painful spasm of the iliocostalis lumborum muscle, a common enough sequel to cystoscopy. But an extra cover had soon warmed her, and Darvon given by mouth relieved her pain. She was due to be discharged next day.

The night nurse coming on duty noticed Mrs. R.'s restless turning about in bed, and pulling at the covers. Perhaps it meant nothing. Her color was good. "How do you feel?" she inquired.

"Oh, all right, I guess," Mrs. R. said, sounding peevish. So the patient was obviously alert. Still, the irritability wasn't a good sign. And now the nurse observed that she was breathing about 30 times a minute and that her skin felt rather warm. Her pulse proved to be 120, her temperature 102° F. Mrs. R. obviously had a good cardiac output because of the flushed, dry, warm skin, and her urinary output had been good. But what about the rapid pulse, hyperventilation, and fever? Adding it all up, the nurse suspected warm shock, a special threat to urological patients.

The deceptive onset of septic shock — warm, dry skin instead of cold, clammy skin; fever instead of subnormal temperatures; normal or excessive urine output instead of oliguria — is one major difference between septic shock and

**Predisposing factors
in septic shock**

TRAUMA AND BURNS. Any injury
that breaks the skin disrupts the
body's defense against
infections.

SURGERY. Peritonitis secondary
to bowel or biliary tract surgery is
a leading cause of septic death.
Surgery of the genitourinary tract
such as transurethral
prostatectomy is another.

INSTRUMENTATION.
Introduction of instruments into
the genitourinary tract, as in
cystoscopy, urethral dilatation, or
bladder catheterization,
frequently induces gram-negative
septicemia because of tissue
trauma or infected urine. Other
major causes of systemic sepsis:
intravascular catheterization
(including I.V. therapy,
hyperalimentation, cardiac
catheterization, pulmonary artery
catheterization, angiography, and
arteriovenous shunts for
hemodialysis), biopsies,
thoracentesis, paracentesis, and
related procedures.

DEFECTS IN HOST RESISTANCE.
Patients with underlying disease
or conditions are particularly
susceptible to septic shock. Be
alert to signs in patients with
diabetes mellitus,
cardiopulmonary insufficiency,
anemias, liver disease, renal
disease, or the like. Carefully
watch the patients undergoing
chemotherapy with
immunosuppressive drugs
(corticosteroids) or
antimetabolites (methotrexate,
fluorouracil, 6-mercaptopurine).

AGE. The newborn's immature
immune system can't combat
respiratory, umbilical, or enteric
infections. The aged's immune
system may not be able to combat
pneumonia, tuberculosis, or even
small, localized infections.

hypovolemic shock. But a second difference is time. In hypovolemic shock, the progression from hypotension to ischemia
to anoxia usually takes several hours — time enough to stop
the bleeding and institute treatment in most patients. In septic
shock, stagnant anoxia may develop in less than an hour —
sometimes in seconds.

Septic patients do eventually develop the classic signs and
symptoms of shock, but by then, their prognosis is very poor.
At best, only 30 to 40% survive; among high-risk patients, only
10% survive.

With the possibility of survival so low, prevention of shock
is far superior to the best treatment. And high on the list of
preventative techniques is assessment and quick action when
early signs of sepsis develop. Your job is to identify your
high-risk patients, to know them well, to recognize early signs
of sepsis, and to begin resuscitation immediately.

Certain patients run far and away the greatest risk of sepsis.
Look for predisposing factors: trauma and burns, surgery,
instrumentation, defects in resistance, infancy or old age, and
superinfections.

Also get to know your patients. You should know them well
enough to detect even subtle deviations from the norm.

This is the key point. Aside from being good nursing practice, knowing your patients gives you the data to make the
preliminary diagnosis of impending septic shock.

Of course, you can't always know every patient well. The
night nurse was scarcely acquainted with Anita R. All that the
night nurse knew of her was what the shift report told her. Still,
like any other urology patient, Mrs. R. was on the high-risk
list, and the nurses well knew it.

If you can, familiarize yourself with the baseline data of all
high-risk patients. That means their admission history, physical exam, lab results. Besides that, get to know their per-
sonalities. And keep an eye on daily assessment data. The
more substantial your data base — your yardstick — the more
easily you can detect even subtle changes in your patient's
behavior. How many septic patients must have been overlooked in the past as being tired, premenstrual, or merely
"having a bad day"?

Recognize the signs of impending septic shock
Classic signs of impending septic shock are:

- restlessness, increasing irritability
- decreasing ability to recall or concentrate, increasing confusion
- loss of consciousness
- faster breathing at greater depth
- higher pulse rate
- abrupt onset of fever (above 101° F.) accompanied by chills and malaise (except in burn patients about to lapse into gram-negative septic shock, who frequently are hypothermic, below 96°)
- sudden, unexplained hypotension (below 80 mm Hg)
- skin that is either warm and dry or cool and clammy
- gastrointestinal symptoms including nausea, vomiting, abdominal cramps, and distention
- blood studies typically show leukopenia, followed by leukocytosis after 6 to 12 hours
- urinalysis shows increased protein and urea nitrogen
- blood gas analysis shows a trend toward metabolic acidosis or, with hyperventilation, alkalosis.

Remember, the patient who is going into septic shock may exhibit only one or two of these signs, not the whole syndrome. (Conversely, a patient showing several of these signs need not be lapsing into septic shock. The signs might be evidence of the original pathology, or of some complication of septicemia other than septic shock.)

Still, you should suspect sepsis in any patient who:
- fits into one or more of the high-risk categories
- exhibits signs of local or septicemia infection
- shows at least one of the classic signs of impending septic shock.

Begin resuscitation...and continue assessment
Septic shock develops so precipitously that resuscitation must be prompt.

In Mrs. R.'s case, the nurse called the resident right away. He asked her to draw blood for arterial gases, to start oxygen at 5 L/min by mask, and to start an I.V. of 1000 cc D₅W.

Why the blood-gas analysis? Because it provides a baseline to determine the adequacy of ventilation and to adjust the concentration of oxygen. Blood gases will be analyzed periodically to find out whether oxygen therapy is effective. Supporting respiration with oxygen is crucial since more septic shock patients die with respiratory problems than with perfusion failure. If the patient remains oliguric and cyanotic despite oxygen and fluid replacement, shunting is likely, and a volume respirator is needed.

Like other kinds of shock, septic shock requires double-barreled treatment: one barrel aimed at the shock; the other at the cause of sepsis. If the focus of infection is known, surgical drainage or administration of the most effective antibiotic should begin immediately.

In the case of Mrs. R., the source of infection was not immediately known, but the resident injected 2 Gms of ampicillin I.V. Within 2 hours, her breathing and pulse had returned to normal; at the end of 12 hours, her white blood count was only slightly elevated.

What was the fulminating infection that had threatened Mrs. R.? It was gram-negative bacteremia cultured as *E. coli,* an ordinarily mild and ever-present bacillus from the intestinal tract. In this case, the septicemia could easily have been caused by its inadvertant surgical introduction through the urinary tract. If you don't know the site of infection, examine your patient from head to toe. Remove and culture all catheters and tubes. But start resuscitation immediately. Too often time that ought to be used to resuscitate the septic patient is wasted while the laboratory checks out a diagnosis.

Patient history: Cardiogenic shock
Margaret A., a 61-year-old postoperative patient had been transferred to the ICU from the surgery unit complaining of chest pain. An EKG showed a possible recent myocardial infarction. The pain was relieved with oxygen and morphine.

One hour after admission, it seemed she had developed sinus tachycardia; pulse, 120/min; blood pressure 95/60.

One of the difficulties in treating cardiogenic shock is that the symptoms of impending shock may be indistinguishable from other conditions. Was Mrs. A. mildly hypotensive because of pain? Because of the morphine? Were there any signs of pulmonary embolus? Of pulmonary edema? What was her temperature? Was septic shock likely? Unfortunately, too, the symptoms of impending cardiogenic shock may be indistinguishable from congestive heart failure. Pulmonary edema; cold, pale, moist extremities; venous distension; and low cardiac output are common to both. You must therefore be par-

POSSIBLE EFFECTS OF VASOCONSTRICTORS		
	EXCESSIVE VASOCONSTRICTION	INADEQUATE VASOCONSTRICTION
Skin color	Pallid or cyanotic	Normal
Skin temperature	Cold	Warm or cool
Pulse	Thready	Good
Blood pressure	Depressed	Depressed
Level of consciousness	Lethargic	Alert
Urinary output	Less than 0.5 cc/min	Less than 0.5 cc/min

ticularly alert to the few signs which distinguish shock from congestive heart failure:

Time. Shock can occur within 30 seconds after an MI or it may develop over a period of hours. Generally, however, its onset is more acute than that of CHF.

Changes in sensorium. Apprehension, confusion, and anxiety in post-MI or cardiac-sugery patients should make you suspicious of either impending shock or pulmonary embolus.

Oliguria. This is more than likely to be a sign of shock than of CHF. It also may indicate renal failure from other causes.

Narrowing of pulse pressure. This is an indication of shock. Blood pressure may drop as much as 30 mm Hg below the patient's normal pressure. Systolic pressure falls before diastolic, producing the narrowed pulse pressure.

Along with a watchful attitude toward signs of cardiogenic shock, you must respond quickly to any changes in the patient's condition that could cause or deepen shock.

Check the patient's pulse frequently and compare it with the apical rate. Report pulse deficits and arrhythmias immediately.

Watch the EKG monitor constantly. Myocardial necrosis, anoxia, and acidosis are fertile soil for the development of arrhythmias.

Check blood gases to make sure you're providing enough oxygen to maintain the PaO_2 between 60 and 90 mm Hg. Most arrhythmias begin at 45, although they may begin with even higher levels in already damaged hearts. High concentrations of oxygen increase peripheral resistance and decrease cardiac output, stroke volume, and heart rate. For this reason, some clinicians recommend maintaining the PaO_2 with large tidal volumes rather than high oxygen concentrations.

At the first sign of shock, increase the oxygen to 100% (7 L/min) and call a physician.

If PAP is not being monitored, watch for dyspnea, cough, rhonchi, or rales, which would indicate pulmonary congestion.

If vasopressors are being given, watch for wide swings in blood pressure and check for fluid overload. Stop the drug immediately and call the physician if signs of overdose develop: headache, chest pain, or frequent premature ventricular contractions.

New monitoring techniques, a better understanding of the pathophysiology of shock, and intelligent use of modern pharmaceutical agents have made some dent in the depressing statistics associated with shock. But none of these advances will work without nurses trained to watch and to interpret what they see.

SKILLCHECK 6

1. Seven-year-old Jennifer Miller was placed on Penicillin-VK 250 mg for a betahemolytic streptococcal throat infection. After her second dose, she complained of abdominal cramps and diarrhea. Mrs. Miller calls the office. What assessments would you tell Mrs. Miller to make?

2. Frank Coletti, a 71-year-old shop owner, was admitted to the CCU with sudden onset of severe, anterior chest pain radiating to both shoulders. On admission, Mr. Coletti was diaphoretic and dyspneic; his blood pressure was 140/80, his pulse 78, and his respirations 12; he had normal sinus rhythm; and he had no signs of congestive heart failure. An EKG and cardiac enzyme levels confirmed a diagnosis of acute anterior-septal MI.

Thirty-six hours after admission, Mr. Coletti had 4 PVCs followed by ventricular tachycardia. You gave 100 mg lidocaine bolus, I.V. push, with 400 watts of countershock. Then you started him on an I.V. infusion of lidocaine 4 mg/min and an I.V. push of propranolol HCl (Inderal) 1 mg. Mr. Coletti converted to sinus rhythm.

In your future assessments of Mr. Coletti, what should you look for?

3. James Polsky, 54 years old, was admitted with burns over 40% of his body from a natural gas explosion. Aggressive fluid replacement and careful monitoring warded off burn shock, and strict isolation techniques were instituted in the hopes of warding off infection.

On his 15th day, Mr. Polsky became mildly febrile and was given acetaminophen (Tylenol) every four hours. By 8 p.m. his blood pressure dropped from 140/80 to 100/70, his urine output decreased, and his CVP dropped to 4 cm H_2O. Feeling that Mr. Polsky was dehydrated, his doctor increased I.V. fluids to 50 ml/hr.

Now, at midnight, Mr. Polsky has become lethargic. His blood pressure is 96/66; respirations, 38 with slight blowing; CVP, 5-6 cm H_2O; temperature 98.6° F. (37° C.). Coughing produces a moderate amount of yellowish sputum. When his blood gas evaluations come back, they read PaO_2, 34; $PaCO_2$, 27; pH, 7.56.

What do you think is happening to Mr. Polsky? What assessments should you make?

4. Lynn Meyer, 25 years old, has been brought to the ER after a car accident. On admission, her neurological functions appear stable, but she is diaphoretic with cool, clammy skin. You take her vital signs: BP, 60/40; pulse, 130; respirations, 40. You find no airway obstruction and no external bleeding. You've noticed marked guarding of her left upper quadrant when you palpate her abdomen, but two consecutive peritoneal taps come out negative. Hemoglobin is a normal 13.5.

What's your assessment?

5. Florence Curry, 68 years old, was admitted with sudden onset of pain in her lower left leg. Her leg appeared mottled, cyanotic, and cool, and her skin was hyperesthetic. The doctor found ischemic ulcers on her toes and no pedal pulses. He diagnosed occlusion of the femoral-popliteal artery and amputated the leg above the knee.

Forty-eight hours post-op, you find Ms. Curry lethargic. When you check her vital signs, you get the following results: BP, 80/50; pulse, thready; respirations, 16; temperature, 100.4° F. (38° C.).

What's your assessment?

(answers on page 186)

SKILLCHECK ANSWERS

ANSWERS TO SKILLCHECK 1 (page 55)

Situation 1 — Emily Jonas
Ms. Jonas' nausea and vomiting could have been caused by two conditions. The first possibility, and most life-threatening, is cardiogenic shock. Other signs of cardiogenic shock include changes in sensorium, narrowing pulse pressure, and oliguria. The second possible cause, and the most likely, is reaction to morphine. Other signs of a reaction include: hypotension, bradycardia, and respiratory depression.

To determine the actual cause, check the color and amount of vomitus and record it as output. Check Ms. Jonas' blood pressure, pulse, respiration, and urinary output. Also check her heart rhythm and, if possible, get an EKG. Finally, note her appearance.

Notify the doctor of your findings and continue to check Ms. Jonas often.

Situation 2 — Mark Schwenk
Even though he doesn't have any clinical symptoms of myocardial infarction, you should check Mr. Schwenk carefully for changes in blood pressure, respiration, color, and pulse. Since the first 24 hours after a myocardial infarction are critical, check his vital signs at least every four hours around the clock. Mr. Schwenk's heart rate of 55/min while awake could easily drop to 38/min during sleep. Although bradycardia may occur normally in athletes, it also can occur after an infarction, in which case it demands prompt treatment to ensure good peripheral perfusion. If Mr. Schwenk's pulse drops markedly during sleep, wake him and begin O₂ therapy (if not already running). Awakening him may provide enough stimulation to raise his respiratory rate. If Mr. Schwenk's heart rate doesn't improve, though, notify the doctor. He may order atropine 0.5 mg I.V. or he may order a temporary pacemaker.

Situation 3 — Sadie and Gwen
Despite their different reactions, both patients probably have pain.

Sadie's pain may be persisting longer than normal because she is anxious about her biopsy, which takes 48 hours to be recorded in her chart. Ask her to describe her pain and the response she gets from medication. If the pain medications help her sleep, she may be using them to escape from her thoughts of cancer.

Because Gwen may be accustomed to the chronic pain of arthritis, she may consider the pain of surgery to be minor. Offer her pain medication, explaining that it will take the edge off her discomfort and help her move better to avoid stiffness and arthritic pain.

Situation 4 — Darlene Brown
Try to determine whether Darlene's problem is pathologic or psychological.

Ask her what is wrong. If she doesn't volunteer information, ask her specific questions:
- Does she feel pain? Is it incisional? If so, give pain medication. If not, try to pinpoint the location. Darlene may be having gas pain; if so, a cup of warm tea and a back rub should take the edge off the pain. A minor tranquilizer, if permitted, can help relax the muscles and lessen the pain.
- Is she worried about her hospitalization? Even though she has coped well until now, she may be suffering from postop depression. She also may be concerned about the surgery, since wedge resections don't guarantee fertility.
- Did a visitor tell her something that makes going home important right now? You may be able to help her work out the problem.

Don't forget the physical aspects of assessment. Check temperature, pulse, respirations, blood pressure, skin around the incision, and intake and output. Any irregularities might indicate infection, or possibly a pulmonary embolus.

Situation 5 — Becky Holz
As you rub Becky's back, note whether she feels discomfort when you touch the raised area. Also note the size, color, and character of the border. Do you find erythema or ulceration?

Ask Becky whether she has noticed the area before. If so, ask when she first noticed it. Find out if she has detected any change in its size or color in the past few months. Also ask if the area feels tender or itchy.

The raised area could be a number of things. It may simply be a congenital condition. Or, it may be an allergic reaction to a drug or to the hospital linen. Or, it could be a skin carcinoma in the very early stage. (Ask Becky if she sunbathes often, since sun exposure contributes to skin carcinoma.)

Suggest that Becky mention the raised area to her doctor the next time he makes rounds. And, if you have the opportunity, mention your assessment to him. Be sure to document your findings and alert the next shift to the condition.

Situation 6 — Rose Serrao

Ask Mrs. Serrao if she has any pain or is anxious about her surgery. If tachycardia and tachypnea persist, investigate further; these signs may indicate incipient heart failure, blood loss, or fat embolism due to long-bone fracture.

Inspect Mrs. Serrao for cyanosis, since sizeable pulmonary emboli always cause hypoxia. Also check for signs of chronic congestive heart failure: engorged neck veins and edema of the leg, ankle, or sacral area.

Check Mrs. Serrao's injured leg for increased swelling, redness, increased warmth; large amounts of blood can leak from an injured blood vessel.

Palpate the liver; tenderness and enlargement, plus a positive hepato-jugular reflex, can indicate right heart failure. Palpate the popliteal and pedal pulses and compare them to pulses in the other leg for signs of arterial occlusion. Also check pulse for regularity; irregularity could be a sign of atrial fibrillation, which often accompanies left heart failure and pulmonary edema. A rapid pulse (over 100) also could indicate heart failure.

Carefully listen to the bases of the lungs for rales or a third heart sound; both are signs of left heart failure. Slight wheezes, too, may occur with early pulmonary edema, especially in an elderly patient. If Mrs. Serrao has pulmonary emboli or pericarditis, you may be able to hear a pleural friction rub over the affected area.

Keep an eye on Mrs. Serrao's level of consciousness, since atherosclerosis, decreased cardiac output, emboli, or hypoxia can dull the sensorium and cause agitation and restlessness.

Notify the doctor of all your findings. Raise the head of Mrs. Serrao's bed to facilitate her breathing, and give O₂ therapy if necessary.

Situation 7 — Alexander Lincoln

Watch Mr. Lincoln for cyanosis. Because of his dark skin, you should check his lips, nailbeds, and palpebral conjunctiva. Don't rely on the color of his gums since many dark-skinned people have a natural bluish tinge to their gums. You also could check Mr. Lincoln's palms; however, if he does manual labor, calluses may interfere with your assessment.

Try to determine whether cyanosis is peripheral or generalized. Generalized cyanosis indicates impaired gas exchange; peripheral cyanosis may indicate low output cardiac failure.

Since cardiogenic shock is always a threat after an infarction, also check for cool, clammy skin when you check for cyanosis. Check for edema of the legs, ankles, and sacral area. If Mr. Lincoln has severe atherosclerosis or mitral valve insufficiency, he may slip into right ventricular failure. Excess fluids then would back up into tissues causing peripheral edema.

When checking Mr. Lincoln's skin, don't limit your assessments to signs of a specific diagnosis. Be sure to check him for other lesions, rashes, and signs of infection or hemorrhage.

ANSWERS TO SKILLCHECK 2 (page 79)

Situation 1 — Mrs. Rasmussen

Inspect the child for signs of increasing cyanosis. Is he breathing at all? Are his respirations labored or shallow? Does his abdomen move up and down with each breath? Do you see intercostal bulging or retraction? If you can, remove any foreign body causing upper airway obstruction. Otherwise, do not waste any time on further questions or examination. Call for help. Time is a critical factor. The brain can't be without oxygen for more than three minutes without irreversible damage, and with an unwitnessed respiratory arrest you have no way of knowing how long the child has been deprived of oxygen.

Situation 2 — Felix Wonder

Looking at Mr. Wonder you would find that his face was purple, that he pursed his lips to breathe, and that his neck veins were distended. His anterior/posterior chest diameter would be increased although both the motion of his diaphragm and his chest expansion would be decreased. When he coughs, he would produce mucus. When palpating you would feel rhonchial fremitus, and when percussing you would hear hyperresonance over his entire chest. During auscultation you would notice distant breath sounds and wheezes, rhonchi, and fine rales in the bases of his lungs. His apical heart sounds would be hard to distinguish. Do not give Mr. Wonder sedation. Call a physician.

Situation 3 — Marty Green

Marty may have a pulmonary embolism. This condition is extremely difficult to diagnose because the clinical picture may vary from tachypnea to chest pain to increasing left ventricular failure to shock. As you inspected Marty you would find her looking anxious; her skin, pale; and her nail beds, blue with slow capillary filling. She would have pleuritic pain, splinting the invalid side, and her respiration would be decreased in depth. When you palpated you would find thready peripheral pulses and sweating. Using the stethoscope you could hear crepitant rales, possibly a friction rub, tachycardia, and a gallop rhythm.

By the way, don't be misled by a normal blood pressure reading; Marty probably has inadequate tissue perfusion and vasoconstriction.

Situation 4 — Peter James

Peter may have a chest contusion or be developing a pneumothorax. Most likely he would appear apprehensive. His buccal membranes would be a normal color, since cyanosis appears only as a late sign of hypoxia, and his neck veins would be distended. Although Peter probably wouldn't have any external signs of injury, you might notice redness over his right ribs. When you palpated, you probably would find tenderness over his right ribs. His trachea would have shifted to the anterior axillary line. You wouldn't find tactile fremitus.

Percussion would reveal hyperresonance. When you auscultated you probably wouldn't hear any breath sounds over the affected area, but you would hear premature heart beats. The presence of hyperresonance and subcutaneous emphysema suggests an internal air leak. In this case you should contact the doctor and administer oxygen, elevating the head of the bed until the physician arrives.

Situation 5 — Joseph Cash
Mr. Cash has uncompensated acute respiratory acidosis with hypoxemia. The normal pH range is 7.35 to 7.45. Mr. Cash's pH is abnormally acidic: 7.2. To determine whether the cause for his acidotic state is respiratory or metabolic, note the respective components of $PaCO_2$ and HCO_3^-. Remember that gases are regulated by the lungs and HCO_3^- is excreted or saved by the kidneys. Plot the three acid-base components pH, $PaCO_2$, and HCO_3^- on the acid-base nomogram. The respective perpendicular lines should converge in the shaded area labeled "acute respiratory acidosis." Since Mr. Cash's oxygen is very low, you can make an accompanying diagnosis of hypoxemia. Some clues from the patient history would support your diagnosis: cessation of ventilation for an undetermined time, questionable respiratory adequacy during resuscitation, and no record of any previous respiratory pathologies.

Situation 6 — Joseph Cash
To obtain the HCO_3^- value, draw a perpendicular line through the marking along the bottom of the nomogram that corresponds to a pH of 7.57. Trace an isobar for a $PaCO_2$ of 25 mm Hg until it connects with the pH line. Lay a ruler perpendicular to this convergent point and draw a line toward the left edge of the nomogram: Mr. Cash's HCO_3^- value is approximately 22 mMol/L.

You will recognize that Mr. Cash has shifted to an uncompensated acute respiratory alkalosis most likely caused by hyperventilation during periods of tachypnea. His hypoxemia resulted from the aeration of one lung. Repositioning the endotracheal tube is imperative.

Situation 7 — Ian Parker
Because of his long smoking history, Mr. Parker has some chronic airway obstruction that predisposes him to hypoventilation after surgery. Knowing this, you should do a thorough chest exam and record your findings. What you need most is an arterial blood-gas report, the most crucial and definitive guide to as-sessment and management. A PaO_2 of less than 50 or a $PaCO_2$ of more than 50 demands immediate attention. In interpreting the gases, recall that his hypoventilation will cause respiratory acidosis due to the CO_2 retention. In Mr. Parker's case, though, the acidosis is likely to be modified by the loss of hydrochloric acid via the nasogastric tube. Loss of HCl without replacement of the chloride ion (Cl^-) produces metabolic alkalosis. The combined result may be a normal or elevated pH in spite of CO_2 retention and a higher-than-normal bicarbonate ion.

ANSWERS TO SKILLCHECK 3 (page 107)

Situation 1 — John Freed
Because of the extensive MI, Mr. Freed is a good candidate for congestive heart failure, which would cause his CVP to rise. But CHF usually drives the CVP way up — as high as 25 cm H_2O. And CVP readings above 10 cm H_2O aren't uncommon in patients with anterior wall infarctions. So, you should assess Mr. Freed for other signs of CHF.

Check his heart rate and rhythm, blood pressure, quality and character of respiration, and vital signs. CHF increases the heart rate and depresses blood pressure. It also may cause rales or a gallop rhythm. As you're bathing Mr. Freed, check for neck vein distention by raising the bed to a 45° angle. Also check his ankles, legs, and sacral area for edema. And check for decreased urinary output.

If you don't find any of these signs of CHF, check the CVP line for a malfunction that would cause the elevated readings. If it is malfunctioning, the readings should return to normal after the doctor changes the catheter. If the CVP line is functioning properly, chances are the anterior wall infarction has produced the slight elevation.

Situation 2 — Marvin Kohn
The decreased urinary output, persistent rales, loud S_3, positive hepatojugular reflex, II/VI holosystolic murmur, and EKG changes — all point to right and left ventricular failure, acute anteroseptal MI, and mitral insufficiency.

Because of Mr. Kohn's decreased cardiac output, Lasix should be continued to remove fluid. Check Mr. Kohn's output carefully, report any increase or decrease, and get frequent serum electrolyte determinations to monitor his potassium depletion, which in excess could cause arrhythmias.

Since Isordil causes vasodilation of the coronary arteries, keep tabs on Mr. Kohn's blood pressure. If it drops, withhold the Isordil and contact the doctor.

Use your auscultory skills to check Mr. Kohn's heart and lungs. Report any changes, such as an increase in rales from the base to scapula, a decrease in breath sounds, or variations in the quality of breath sounds and heart sounds.

Because venous return to the heart is elevated, you should watch Mr. Kohn closely for signs of shortness of breath, dyspnea, or increased heart rate.

And, because his cardiac output and possible tissue perfusion is depressed, you should frequently check Mr. Kohn's skin color and skin warmth for signs of ischemia and possible skin breakdown.

Situation 3 — Karen Porter
You should have closely monitored Mrs. Porter's vital signs, blood pressure, heart rhythm, and intake and output for any signs of heart failure, which can easily follow an infarction.

You also should have checked her CVP line for proper infusion and patency, and you should have checked the insertion site for signs of infection (redness, swelling, tenderness, or a foul smell). When taking a reading, you should have made sure that Mrs. Porter was supine and that the manometer was level with her atrium at the midaxillary line. (Although Mrs. Porter's CVP readings remained stable, you should have expected her respirations to cause some fluctuation, about 2 cm.)

Situation 4 — Mr. Barker
The EKG changes and elevation of serial enzymes indicate acute anterior wall infarction. Changes in blood pressure and pulse, the presence of an S_3 gallop rhythm and rales, a decrease to less than 30 cc of urinary output per hour, and an increase in PAP — all point to heart failure with decreased cardiac output.

You should take Mr. Barker's vital signs frequently, along with PAP and PWP readings and hourly urinary outputs. Immediately report any change.

Check Mr. Barker's radial and brachial pulses, as well as the color and temperature of his arm; decreased pulses, cyanosis, and coolness could indicate that a hematoma from the Swan-Ganz cutdown is occluding the artery.

Watch the oscilloscope for proper pulmonary artery tracings. If the tracing disappears or becomes erratic, check for a blood return. If you don't get one, the catheter may be stranded in the wedge position, a clot may have formed at the catheter's end, the catheter may be damped along the wall of the pulmonary artery, or the balloon may have ruptured. If the balloon has ruptured (no resistance on irrigation) or you can't aspirate an obstruction, notify the doctor immediately.

Continue O_2 therapy and watch the cardiac monitor for arrhythmias.

Situation 5 — Pat Sell
Look for neck vein distention and atrial or ventricular arrhythmias. Without a CVP, these signs would be your first clues to fluid overload and would develop before hypotension and narrow pulse pressure.

Look, too, for edema of the legs, ankles, and sacral area, particularly if Pat's urinary output decreases significantly. Although a drop in urinary output can indicate hypovolemia, it also can indicate lack of renal perfusion, which causes more fluid retention.

Routinely listen to Pat's heart and breath sounds. If you hear a gallop rhythm or rales, report them to the doctor and check Pat's condition more often.

When checking Pat's pulse rate, remember that she is on Digoxin, which decreases pulse rate. Find out from the doctor what Pat's rate should be; it might range anywhere from 60 to 120.

ANSWERS TO SKILLCHECK 4 (page 127)

Situation 1 — Ralph Reeder
Mr. Reeder would have pain radiating from his back or side across his abdomen and into his groin, genitalia, or inner thigh. Unlike patients with intraperitoneal inflammation who lie very still, Mr. Reeder probably would make writhing movements.

You would find slight tenderness over the involved kidney and ureter and you might find spasms of the abdominal muscles. Urinalysis would show albuminuria and hematuria (usually only in microscopic amounts).

Situation 2 — Bob Blackmore
Compare total intake (including I.V. fluids) to total output. Perhaps Mr. Blackmore is being held NPO in preparation for a test. Or he may be losing fluids in other ways, through fever, vomiting, diarrhea, diaphoresis, hyperventilation, or wound drainage. Check his chart to make sure he isn't taking any medications that might cause urinary retention. Also ask other nurses on the floor if they've noticed output that may not have been charted.

Since congestive heart failure is a possibility, check Mr. Blackmore's blood pressure and pulse to see if they're markedly decreased. Also listen to his heart for S_3 or S_4 sounds. Check urine for an elevated specific gravity (over 1.030).

Also, check Mr. Blackmore's skin for turgor, dryness, firmness, clamminess, and edema.

No matter what your findings, record them, notify the doctor, and keep a close watch on Mr. Blackmore's output and general condition.

Situation 3 — Pam Galt
Ask Pam to describe her symptoms more fully: How long has she had the burning? Is it accompanied by frequency or urgency? Does she have a fever? Does her urine contain blood? Does she have nausea and vomiting? Diarrhea? Abdominal pain? Back pain?

The most likely explanation for Pam's burning sensation is cystitis, a common complication of diabetes. Ask Pam if she's ever had urinary tract infections. If so, how frequently and how were they treated? This information, along with details on any medications she might be taking, will help the doctor identify and treat her problem.

Situation 4 — Vincent Douglas

Chances are Mr. Douglas would appear pallid, with cool, clammy skin. He would have respiratory difficulties and, if his diaphragm had ruptured, he would be using his abdominal muscles to breathe. He would feel tenderness over the left lateral rib cage and pain in the left upper quadrant and left shoulder. Spasm and tenderness also might extend down to his pelvis because of the irritation caused by extravasated blood. Adjacent organs such as the stomach and splenic flexure of the colon would be displaced away from the left upper quadrant. His urine also might contain blood for internal bleeding.

Because of his internal blood loss, you should check Mr. Douglas for signs of hypovolemic shock (see next section). You also should check for dyspnea, rales, decreased cardiac output, and possibly S_3 and S_4 heart sounds, all of which would indicate congestive heart failure.

Situation 5 — Marlene Jacobs

You probably would notice some ataxia and asterixis. You might find small spider angiomas on Ms. Jacob's body, particularly around her face, due to capillary fragility. The skin on her abdomen would appear smooth and thick, with striae. In addition to abdominal distention, she probably would have bulging flanks.

If you auscultated Ms. Jacob's abdomen, you would hear bowel sounds. Because of the ascites, percussion would elicit dullness in the midabdomen when Ms. Jacob was standing, her flank area when she lay down, and her dependent side when she rolled onto her side. If you palpated from the midaxillary line on the right side, you probably would find the liver enlarged with a firm, irregular edge.

Situation 6 — Joan Rodriquez

Mrs. Rodriguez probably would be jaundiced, particularly in the sclera and nailbeds. Her respiration and chest movement during respiration probably would be normal. But her pulse and CBC would be elevated. If she had intestinal obstruction, you might hear hypoactive bowel sounds on auscultation.

When palpating, you probably would find spasms of the right rectus abdominus and flank muscle, with rebound tenderness. You also might find pain in the right upper quadrant that periodically would radiate to her back up to the scapula.

Situation 7 — Daniella Brown

Usually in appendicitis, the patient lies on his side with his knees flexed near his abdomen. Daniella's abdomen probably wouldn't be distended unless the appendix ruptured, causing a contained, local abscess.

If the appendix had ruptured several hours before, you probably would notice gaseous distention.

Auscultation probably would reveal hypoactive or no bowel sounds. Daniella might complain of pain around the umbilicus initially and later of pain in the lower right quadrant. She also would have rebound and percussion tenderness at McBurney's point. (If you percussed other areas of Daniella's abdomen or if she coughed, pain would refer to McBurney's point.) Daniella also would have spasms of the lower abdominal muscles on her right side.

You would expect Daniella's temperature and CBC to be elevated. If the appendix had ruptured and caused peritonitis, you would find an elevated pulse and a rising temperature.

ANSWERS TO SKILLCHECK 5 (page 149)

Situation 1 — Mark Banner

The slow pulse, elevated blood pressure, and wide pulse pressure all point to an increase in intracranial pressure. Try to establish an open airway by correctly positioning Mark's head, making sure his tongue hasn't fallen back in his throat, and inserting an oral or nasal airway. Notify his doctor immediately.

Situation 2 — John Cannon

There seem to be two problems here. On one hand, the downward change in John's level of consciousness, movement, and pupil responses, maybe from bleeding or cerebral edema. Since increased intracranial pressure creates a potentially dangerous situation, you should notify John's doctor and make cranial checks more often to detect further changes.

On the other hand, though, the changes in blood pressure and pulse are typical of hypovolemic shock rather than increased intracranial pressure. Since an adult couldn't have enough cranial bleeding to account for these symptoms, you should look for other sources of injury and bleeding. Report your findings to John's doctor and continue to monitor him.

Situation 3 — Pattie O'Dell

This is a matter of judgment. Since Pattie's accident occurred recently and since intracranial pressure can increase suddenly, you probably should continue frequent cranial checks. Pattie's irritation at being awakened may or may not be a symptom of concussion or increased intracranial pressure. If it isn't, her irritation will probably subside if you explain how important the cranial checks are.

Situation 4 — Susan

Susan's behavior — the headaches and lethargy — aren't normal for a 4-year-old, or for an adult either. These symptoms may have nothing to do with Susan's fall. But they could indicate increased intracranial pressure from a subdural hematoma that has been slowly developing since her fall. No matter what the cause, advise Susan's mother to take Susan to a doctor as soon as possible for further evaluation.

Situation 5 — George Williams

Since a change in level of consciousness may be the first sign of increasing intracranial pressure, you should suspect increased pressure, probably as a result of the subarachnoid hemorrhage. Chances are Mr. Williams was straining while using the bedpan, causing Valsalva's maneuver. The elevated intrathoracic pressure would have been transmitted directly to the brain, raising the intracranial pressure.

Look for other signs of increased intracranial pressure. The pupil on Mr. William's affected side would be dilated and fixed. His pulse and respiration would be decreased, while his blood pressure would have risen.

Call the doctor immediately. Remember that massive subarachnoid hemorrhages often cause respiratory arrest and herniation of the brain through the tentorial notch, ending in death.

ANSWERS TO SKILLCHECK 6 (page 179)

Situation 1 — Jennifer Miller

Allergic reactions may produce acute circulatory failure (anaphylaxis) without warning or with prodromal signs such as fever, diarrhea, abdominal cramps, or rash. Tell Mrs. Miller to stop giving the penicillin. Then, ask her to check Jennifer for hives on her face, trunk, or legs; facial swelling; or breathing difficulties. If Mrs. Miller has diphenhydramine HCl (Benadryl) elixir, have her give Jennifer 1-2 teaspoons immediately. If Jennifer's symptoms subside, the doctor will prescribe another antibiotic. If Jennifer's symptoms persist or worsen, however, Mrs. Miller should immediately take her to the doctor's office or to the hospital emergency room for possible emergency treatment.

Situation 2 — Frank Coletti

Cardiac patients with severe recurring complications such as tachycardia are predisposed to cardiogenic shock. So, you should monitor Mr. Coletti closely. Watch him for early signs of shock, such as dehydration, decreased urinary output, change in level of consciousness, decreased blood pressure, rapid and thready pulse, or cardiac arrhythmias.

Also check for signs of fluid overload, such as gallop heart sounds, neck-vein distention, positive hepatojugular reflex, rales in lung fields, and edema of the leg, sacrum, or foot. Monitor Mr. Coletti's vital signs and urinary output frequently; document and report any changes. Make sure that O_2 therapy and emergency equipment are readily available.

Situation 3 — James Polsky

Mr. Polsky is showing signs of pulmonary congestion and oxygen desaturation. Probable cause: septic shock. In fact, he probably was in septic shock when the doctor first suspected dehydration. But septic shock is difficult to diagnose in the early stages. The most reliable signs are hyperventilation and decreased blood pressure, CVP, and urine output.

Besides recognizing and treating the shock, you should look for the cause of the sepsis. Get a culture of blood, wounds, urine, sputum, and spinal fluid. Chances are Mr. Polsky has sepsis of the pulmonary system (including the nasopharynx), burn wounds, or urinary tract. But he may have an infection of the cerebral ventricles, caused by organisms entering through his burn wounds.

Monitor Mr. Polsky's status, frequently checking pulse, temperature, respiration, CVP, blood pressure, and urinary output. Also check his level of consciousness and *Stat* report restlessness or agitation. Every 4 hours, make a cranial check — motor function, pupil size, and level of consciousness. Also check the skin around I.V. lines for signs of sepsis — redness, tenderness, changes in skin temperature, or swelling.

Situation 4 — Lynn Meyer

Despite normal hemoglobin, Ms. Meyer clearly is in hypovolemic shock. She needs constant monitoring and aggressive management to restore blood volume.

Frequently check her CVP, blood pressure, pulse, pulse pressure (systolic minus diastolic), and urine output to make sure her I.V. infusion rate is adequate without being excessive.

Ms. Meyer should have another peritoneal tap to check for gross blood, a sign of internal bleeding. (Splenic rupture and other causes of internal bleeding are fairly common in trauma patients.)

With fluid replacement and correction of any fluid loss, Ms. Meyer should fully recover.

Situation 5 — Florence Curry

Any of these findings in a postsurgical patient should alert you to septic shock. Call the doctor; draw blood for gases; start oxygen; and start an I.V.

In Ms. Curry's case, the cause of septic shock could well be gangrene. You would recognize it by foul-smelling fluid and gas escaping from the stump and a mushy appearance. If lab reports confirmed the diagnosis, the doctor would probably amputate further and start the patient on antibiotics, antitoxins, and steroid therapy. After the second surgery, monitor urinary drainage and vital signs to pick up early signs of recurrent shock. Also check the stump for bright red bleeding. Outline the original drainage on the dressing with a pen and immediately report any increase to the doctor.

Remember, too, that elderly postsurgical patients on bedrest are prone to pulmonary emboli. Remember the signs: a sharp, stabbing pain in the chest; breathlessness with cyanosis; pupil dilation; cold sweating; and rapid, irregular, diminishing pulse.

INDEX